completely
normal
and
totally
fine

completely normal and totally fine

My Life with Bipolar Disorder

rosie viva

TONIC
LONDON · OXFORD · NEW YORK · NEW DELHI · SYDNEY

BLOOMSBURY TONIC
Bloomsbury Publishing Plc
50 Bedford Square, London, WC1B 3DP, UK
Bloomsbury Publishing Ireland Limited,
29 Earlsfort Terrace, Dublin 2, D02 AY28, Ireland

BLOOMSBURY, BLOOMSBURY TONIC and the Tonic logo are trademarks of
Bloomsbury Publishing Plc

First published in Great Britain 2025
Copyright © Rosie Viva, 2025

Rosie Viva is identified as the author of this work in accordance with the
Copyright, Designs and Patents Act 1988.

All rights reserved. No part of this publication may be: i) reproduced or transmitted in any form, electronic or mechanical, including photocopying, recording or by means of any information storage or retrieval system without prior permission in writing from the publishers; or ii) used or reproduced in any way for the training, development or operation of artificial intelligence (AI) technologies, including generative AI technologies. The rights holders expressly reserve this publication from the text and data mining exception as per Article 4(3) of the Digital Single Market Directive (EU) 2019/790

Bloomsbury Publishing Plc does not have any control over, or responsibility for, any third-party websites referred to in this book. All internet addresses given in this book were correct at the time of going to press. The author and publisher regret any inconvenience caused if addresses have changed or sites have ceased to exist, but can accept no responsibility for any such changes

A catalogue record for this book is available from the British Library

ISBN: HB: 978-1-5266-7942-0; eBook: 978-1-5266-7941-3;
ePDF: 978-1-5266-7940-6

2 4 6 8 10 9 7 5 3 1

Typeset by Newgen KnowledgeWorks Pvt. Ltd., Chennai, India

Printed and bound in Great Britain by Clays Ltd, Elcograf S.p.A.

To find out more about our authors and books visit www.bloomsbury.com
and sign up for our newsletters

For product safety related questions contact
productsafety@bloomsbury.com

To my mum, Amanda, and dad, Victor, for believing in my return to Rosie.

CONTENTS

	Introduction	1
1	Before everything changed	7
2	Going south	19
3	Unravelling	33
4	Detached from reality	49
5	Hello darkness, my old friend	69
6	The bumpy road to recovery	89
7	Rediscovering Rosie	103
8	The light behind trauma	113
9	Finding my voice	127
10	Loving (and losing) with bipolar	147
11	My mind at work	167
12	Riding the ups and downs	183
13	Give yourself time	199
	Our voices	211
	Acknowledgements	217

DISCLAIMER

While this is a first-hand account of a bipolar 1 diagnosis, sharing my personal experience and opinions on the topic, I am not a clinical psychologist or psychiatrist. This book should not be a substitute for medical advice. Please always consult a medical professional before considering any change in your lifestyle. This book mentions suicide, self-harm and other scenarios you may find triggering.

For readers seeking further information or support regarding bipolar disorder, Bipolar UK is a valuable resource. They provide expert advice, support services and a community for individuals living with bipolar disorder, as well as their families and carers. You can access more information and support on their website at www.bipolaruk.org.

introduction

Over the past few years, my life has been the opposite of 'normal'.

Needing my mum to tuck me into bed every night, at the age of twenty-three?

Not normal.

Believing I have been chosen by God?

Not normal.

Jumping through oversized baggage in an airport and setting off the fire alarm?

Not even *slightly* normal.

Sitting in a circle banging on African drums with a group of mentally ill strangers?

Anything *but* normal.

Welcome to my life.

Before 2018, I would have told you that everything was just fine. In fact, it was more than fine – it was undeniably great. I had an amazing job as a model, which enabled me to work with huge brands and travel the world. I had a buzzing social life and a fun, loving relationship with my boyfriend. Sure, I suffered from the occasional bout of anxiety and depression, but that's par for the course when you're in your teens and early twenties, right?

My life turned upside down when I experienced an intense manic episode – a psychotic breakdown in which I hallucinated vividly and lived on another planet (under lock and key in a mental health ward) for almost three months straight. This led to my diagnosis of bipolar disorder, which I'd likely had for a few years without realising it. In the years since leaving hospital, I've been navigating the highs and lows (literally) that my illness brings; sometimes going in the right direction, sometimes going off-track, and sometimes going around and around in circles until I'm back where I started.

Bipolar disorder (formerly known as manic depression) is a mental health condition that affects your moods, and while it might not be considered 'normal', it is actually surprisingly common. Recent figures from the National Institute for Health and Care Excellence (NICE) suggest about 2 per cent of the population in the UK has a bipolar diagnosis (which equates to roughly 1.5 million people).[1] There's a relatively even split between men and women, and the average age of onset is twenty-five years old (three years older than I was when I was diagnosed). It's so common that most people probably know someone who has bipolar, even if they don't quite understand what it means, or the impact it can have.

I know people often describe unpredictable weather as 'bipolar'. It doesn't annoy me when people use the word so flippantly in this way, because it's actually true. Bipolar is

---

[1] Bipolar disorder: How common is it? NICE Clinical Knowledge Summaries, last revised April 2024. https://cks.nice.org.uk/topics/bipolar-disorder/background-information/incidence-prevalence

just like British weather, in particular. Up and down, unreliable and often extreme. One day, you wake up and the sun is streaming through the windows: everything seems perfect and beautiful, and like nothing could ever go wrong. That's the equivalent of hypomania – or 'highs' – which is a key sign of bipolar. Hypomanic periods are characterised by euphoria, high energy, optimism that can easily cross over into delusion, and risky or impulsive behaviour.

Then, just as you go outside to bask in the sun, it starts to rain – hard. The sky turns completely black, seemingly absorbing all the good in the world, ruining all your plans and all your excitement. The blustery wind hits your face, and all you want to do is run back inside and huddle under your duvet indefinitely. That's the equivalent of depression – another sign of bipolar: low periods that feel empty, pointless and dark.

While many mental health conditions involve depression, you're likely to be diagnosed with bipolar if you switch between both kinds of extreme mood on a relatively regular basis. Low and high periods can last for minutes, days, weeks or months, depending on the type of bipolar and the individual. Again, just like the British weather.

However, what many people don't know about bipolar is that it is divided into two separate diagnoses. Bipolar 2 consists of hypomania and depression. In bipolar 1, hypomania has the potential to escalate into full-blown mania, otherwise known as psychosis. This is one of the most feared and stigmatised symptoms in any mental health condition, because sufferers completely lose their grip on reality. This can be extremely dangerous but is normally only dangerous to the person experiencing it.

During my manic episode, I didn't really know what was going on. It was scarier for my loved ones watching me talk nonsense about monkeys and run around the hospital corridors removing various articles of clothing. For me, the trauma of that incident, and the deep, dark depression that followed, was the scariest part. It's estimated that between 25 per cent and 60 per cent of people with bipolar will attempt suicide at least once in their life, and between 4 per cent and 9 per cent will complete it.[2]

I know that all sounds pretty terrifying, and to be honest, I get it. When my medication brought me back down to earth, my diagnosis initially felt like a death sentence. I didn't know anyone else who had bipolar. It didn't help that all the accounts I read about the condition came from people I couldn't relate to, who spoke of repeated psychotic breakdowns and suicide. No wonder so much stigma about bipolar (and mental health) remains, when we often talk about it in such gruesome negative terms (if we talk about it at all). I genuinely believed my life would be filled with chaos, depression and mania – on loop – forever and ever.

My journey with bipolar hasn't been easy, and it has certainly been one of extreme highs and extreme lows. But it hasn't always been the hellish road I was led to believe it would be. Since my diagnosis, I have fallen in love (and out of it), changed career direction (several times) and switched medications and treatments (more times than I can count) until I finally found what works for me. In learning more about my illness, I have directed my energy towards speaking out about mental health, and I even made a documentary called 'Modelling, Mania and Me', which aired on Channel 4 in 2023.

---

[2] Dome P, Rihmer Z and Gonda X, 'Suicide Risk in Bipolar Disorder: A Brief Review', *Medicina (Kaunas)*, vol. 55(8): page 403, 2019. doi: 10.3390/medicina55080403. https://www.ncbi.nlm.nih.gov/pmc/articles/PMC6723289/

While making the documentary – and in the months that followed – I heard from so many more people like me. Young people who had no idea what they were experiencing or how to manage their moods, and who were getting through each day with a lot of trial and error. Discovering this community has been so heartwarming and invigorating. Knowing that other people have been through similar experiences and still manage to live fulfilling lives has made me feel so much less alone. Finding a community of normal people with abnormal minds has been incredible and affirming.

So, that's why I decided to write this book. Conversations about mental health have been opening up over the years thanks to amazing spokespeople, from writers such as Matt Haig and Bryony Gordon to sports stars and high-profile names such as Simone Biles and Naomi Osaka. It's so important for us to speak up about mental health, so that other people gain a better understanding of this condition that affects so many, and sadly takes so many lives.

I wanted to write this book for every young person who has felt hopeless and lost because of a mental health diagnosis. I want you to know that there *are* better days ahead. I'll be honest: the rocky road of recovery has included numerous heartbreaks and failures. Bipolar is a serious mental health condition and shouldn't be taken lightly. But there has also been a huge amount of love, connection, joy and genuine hilarity. It's not all doom and gloom, I promise.

With that in mind, we should probably go back to the beginning.

1
before everything changed

Alongside my tattoos ('Monday' and 'Life is weird'), I have often thought about getting the year '2018' inked somewhere on my body. It was a bizarre year, not least because it was the year I hurtled towards a psychotic episode, was sectioned and was then diagnosed with bipolar 1.

Sometimes, I cast my mind back over my life before that time and try to look for warning signs. It's potentially a pointless exercise, because hindsight is a wonderful thing, and it's also normal to have fluctuating moods and struggles when you're a child or teen. It can be difficult to know where my personality ends and bipolar begins. Still, I think it's important to go back to the very start.

I was born in West London and spent my early years living in Hammersmith with my parents – who ran an advertising company together – and my two older sisters, Amii and Lucy. Before I was born, my parents had lost a son, Alex, to leukaemia when he was seven years old. I'd always known about the tragic loss of the brother I'd never met, but my parents are the most positive people you'll ever meet. The trauma encouraged them to live every day like it's their last, and they instilled that in us too.

If you asked my mum what I was like as a child, the first thing she'd say is how sensitive I was. I cried all the time (I still do) and felt hugely attached to her, leading the rest of the family to call me 'clingy'. I wanted to do everything with her, even if she was just going to the shops or doing household chores. It was as if I was her shadow, and I became jealous whenever she gave attention to my sisters rather than to me. Case in point: she had to give me presents on Amii and Lucy's birthdays, as otherwise I'd feel left out.

I think this is normal when you're the youngest child, right? I was the baby, and my sisters treated me as such. My middle sister, Lucy, knew how much I craved everyone's attention, so her favourite way to wind me up was to completely ignore me. When I tried to speak with her, she'd pretend I wasn't even there. It felt like torture, as if she was looking through me, and I'd find it so distressing that I'd end up running to my mum in tears.

I needed a lot of comfort and reassurance as a child and insisted on being tucked into bed when I was probably too old to need that. I wanted to sleep in my parents' bed until I was about five years old, and would often bang on their door screaming until they'd let me in. I wasn't the kind of child who could just be left alone to their own devices. My sisters would wander off and read or play by themselves. I found that borderline impossible. I always needed to be around people, hovering and wanting to be involved with whatever they were doing.

When I was seven, my parents decided they wanted to raise us outside the city, so we moved to the countryside in Gloucestershire, with my parents commuting into London.

I was young, so it didn't feel like a dramatic move to me. I wasn't really attached to anyone or anything beyond my parents and sisters, so wherever they went, I was happy to follow. As I had always loved being outside in nature, moving somewhere with a proper garden seemed exciting – plus my parents had promised that we could get a pet rabbit. Moving into our new house and going to a new school felt like a big adventure.

Like a lot of young girls who are loud, I was known at school for being 'bossy'. I was used to being described like this at home too. I was known for always wanting to be in control, and Lucy hated that I always had strong opinions about whatever she did. At school, I was the typical snitch, telling on my classmates if it meant the teachers would like me. I even wrote to Tony Blair (the then Prime Minister) to tell him about a girl at school who fox hunted. I really believed I would get a response from Tony. Perhaps this was the start of my grand ideas, which would later become a defining feature of my hypomanic episodes. Or maybe I was simply an imaginative child. A few years later, I wrote to the White House during the war in Afghanistan. I sent a letter in the post, with the lyrics to 'Where Is The Love?' by the Black Eyed Peas. Shockingly, I didn't receive a response.

When I started secondary school, the 'bossy' label stuck. My school was divided into boarders and day students. I was a day student because we only lived around the corner. But, given I always wanted to be involved and included, I hated how all my friends had sleepovers every night and I had to go home. So when I was in Year 8, I convinced my parents to let me board. I loved it and, funnily enough, it made me a lot more independent. I lost that clinginess to my parents, and instead threw myself into life with my friends.

I was known for my sense of humour, which I wore like a badge of honour. I loved to say things people didn't expect and make them laugh. Whether it was challenging a teacher or being in the centre of a group of girls, I made a point of being sarcastic or self-deprecating and embarrassing myself.

Despite being the class clown, I was still extremely sensitive. When I was fifteen, a friend of mine developed anorexia. As a result, I began to stop eating properly. I've always been a sponge, taking on whatever is going on with other people around me. During that period, I was so distressed by my friend's illness, seeing her faint and, later on, having to quit school altogether. I struggled to concentrate on my schoolwork because I was so preoccupied with how she was doing. Watching her physically change so much, and seeing how worried all the adults were, made me anxious, afraid and distracted. It's easy to link my extreme reaction to bipolar now, but at the time everyone just thought I was a bit delicate.

Around this time, my first boyfriend (a cool, indie boy who played guitar) dumped me. My parents were worried about how everything was affecting me, so on my suggestion they agreed to send me to a different boarding school for my A-levels. In reality, I was just running away from unhappiness, which is obviously impossible to do.

This was the year I began to hide what was going on with my mental health. I knew I was going downhill, but I realised that as long as I continued smiling and making people laugh, nobody would suspect a thing. I think this is still the case twelve years later. I've always dealt with a confused mind by projecting joy to everyone else.

These years weren't all bad. It was during this time that I started modelling, which would go on to change the course of my life. I became obsessed with the idea of modelling when my first boyfriend (the one who dumped me) began dating a model straight after me (that'll show him!). I was desperate to get scouted, and I'd heard that you needed to hang around in Central London waiting to be spotted by a model scout. So in my school holidays, I'd go with my friends to Oxford Circus with heeled boots on, flicking my hair around, hoping someone in the industry would think I was gorgeous and decide to give me a shot.

The rumours were right, but it happened when I least expected it. I was randomly walking through Camden Market with a friend when a scout approached me and asked if I had ever tried modelling. I was thrilled. The woman gave me her card and asked me to come in for a meeting. I immediately called my mum to tell her the good news. Fortunately, my parents were relaxed and happy for me to get on with it. I went off to agencies and castings in my school holidays, and before I knew it I had landed a summer teen edit campaign for a well-known supermarket chain. The campaign hit shop floors as soon as I started sixth form, and it was a major hit of validation. I felt so smug with my thousands of Facebook friends (a real status symbol in Gloucestershire at the time) who would leave comments such as 'Stunning xxx' on every picture (my mum commented too, but I deleted those).

When I finished school, I was offered a university place at University College London to study history of art and material sciences. Lucy had been to UCL, and she's known to be a genius, so my logic for applying was along the lines of, 'If I go to UCL, it'll show that I am a genius too.' My A-level results were good, but what I really excelled in was philosophy, scoring 100 per cent on my exams. I was obsessed with the subject and didn't really care about the others, to be honest. I was hooked, spending hours reading around the topics we had studied in class, listening to countless talks and clocking in extra time with my teacher. By contrast, I found geography pointless and couldn't put any energy into it, and that reflected in my grades. I'm still this way now. If I'm interested in something, I can become hyper-focused. But if I'm not, I struggle to focus at all. I just knew that whichever direction I followed, a meander bend wasn't something I'd be talking about ever again beyond school. So why would a good grade in this subject help me?

I soon realised that I didn't really want to go to university – I just wanted to get in. I thought about my experiences of education and realised that the environment didn't suit me. I hated being told what to do and couldn't imagine more years of that. With my modelling career burgeoning, I decided *this* was what I wanted to do full-time, so I deferred my university place and decided to throw myself completely into modelling.

The summer after I finished school, I moved back to London so I could go to more castings. It was during this time that my mum became worried about me. I was sleeping all the time, feeling low, and I was constantly lacking in energy. Mum marched me off to the doctor. I was diagnosed with an underactive thyroid (where your thyroid gland doesn't produce enough hormones, resulting in fatigue, depression and other physical symptoms from weight gain to constipation). I was told that this was the cause of my lifelessness (a massive relief), and I was prescribed medication to take long-term to support my thyroid and boost my energy levels.

I didn't think too deeply about this diagnosis at the time – I was just pleased to have an answer (and solution) for how

I'd been feeling. For the whole of sixth form, I would say I was hiding depression, so a doctor implying that this new medication would fix that was exciting. But I now know that bipolar disorder is often misdiagnosed in women as an underactive thyroid and the two conditions are closely linked. Multiple studies[1] have suggested that people with bipolar are more likely to have thyroid issues than the general population, although it's hard to know if one is the cause and the other is the effect. Either way, there's a correlation between the two conditions that isn't talked about enough. But we'll come back to that later.

The medication seemed to work a treat. I was suddenly bursting with energy. My excitement for life was huge, and I wanted to be out all day and night with friends, enjoying my new-found freedom. That said, my first year out of school was the biggest flop ever. I began working with a prestigious modelling agency that represented huge names such as Kendall Jenner. But they didn't send me to many castings, and I didn't work once. Instead, I spent the majority of my time clubbing in Mayfair with promoters and generally being really cringe. My parents, unsurprisingly, weren't too happy about it and reminded me I still had my place at UCL. But I still loved modelling, so I pleaded, telling them I'd find a new agency. They agreed to give me one more year to turn things around.

Fortunately, my luck took a turn. The first job my new agency found for me was with Saint Laurent in Paris. I know that sounds very glamorous, but I was a 'fittings model', which basically just means you're a living mannequin for

---

[1]Chakrabarti S, 'Thyroid functions and bipolar affective disorder', *Journal of Thyroid Research*, 306367, 2011. https://doi.org/10.4061/2011/306367 https://pubmed.ncbi.nlm.nih.gov/21808723/

them to put clothes on and see how everything looks during the designing process. I showed up on the casting day wearing the most ridiculous emo-chic outfit, trying to look like a quintessential 'Saint Laurent girl'.

Looking around at all the beautiful models, I didn't think it was likely I'd get the job. But they didn't take any pictures, only my measurements (including the size of my head). It turns out I was perfect for what they were looking for, as my measurements were the closest to one of their dress sizes. I accepted the job and began working the very next day.

That contract lasted for six months – pretty rare, considering most modelling roles aren't consistent or well-paid. However, it was extremely lonely. I had moved to Paris on my own and was renting a small studio apartment, working with people who didn't speak English and didn't even bother learning my name. Everyone kept telling me I was doing *so* well. I was nineteen and earning great money, meaning I could save up to purchase a flat, and I was getting my name out there in the modelling world. But deep down, I felt so low. Even worse, feeling that way made me think I was being ungrateful. I would never have said the word 'depression' out loud.

Modelling is a funny old business, and it's sort of unsurprising that my mental health issues spiralled in this time. I sometimes wonder whether I would have developed bipolar had I chosen to go to uni and lived a more stable, routine existence in that precious period between the ages of eighteen and twenty-two (which is when bipolar is most likely to develop). The exact causes of bipolar still aren't understood. However, experts believe environmental factors can increase the likelihood of developing it.

There was an immense amount of pressure on my appearance. After my contract in Paris and a few other jobs in London, and still only nineteen years old, I set off for the bright lights of New York City. My agency promised that I could be the 'next big model' on the runway shows, but warned that if my hips got bigger than 34", I would be sent home, unable to cast. I had been into running since school – to this day, it's my favourite form of escape and clarity – but I was running more than ever, desperately trying to keep myself small for my high-fashion moment. After securing the biggest job of my life – I walked a show for Gucci – I thought I'd achieved my big break. But, unfortunately, no other casting directors saw me as the next big star, so my agency advised me to start working in the commercial world instead.

Not long after this disappointment, I booked my first commercial job for a large fashion brand for a ridiculous amount of money. It was a dream client for my new direction, as it was a brand that all my friends were wearing at the time, and everything was finally starting to look up. My New York days were full of energy and exuberance. I began living with a friend in Brooklyn and threw myself into exercising (sometimes twice a day) and going out (all day and all night).

My life went from 'normal' to 'perfect' in a heartbeat. The sky seemed to always be bright and blue, and I became obsessed with exploring the city. I would even walk back from castings that were hours away, just so I could mooch around different neighbourhoods and take everything in. It felt as if anything was possible. I was constantly meeting new people during the day and then partying with them at night, in clubs and house parties all around New York.

Modelling in the US was a whole different world too: you were treated like royalty on set. Every time someone was sent to fetch a coffee for me, I felt as if I was the main character in a movie. The rates were also mind-blowing. I was young and earning more than I had ever made – it was quite a lot to ingest. Everyone around me (including my family and friends back home) were telling me how *well* I was doing, and I was swept up in the fantasy of it all. *This is what people dream of!* I thought, almost every day. *This is everything YOU have dreamed of!*

It's hard to look back on the rose-tinted memories of this time in my life and think, *Oh yes, that was the bipolar kicking off*. But I now know that hypomania – periods of overactive and high-energy behaviour that dramatically impact your everyday life, usually over a short period of time – can be beautiful. I didn't think I was having any problems with my mental health. We've always been taught that feeling positive is a good thing; we're not trained to think of it as a warning sign. Plus, my hyper personality fitted in perfectly with American culture. I was always referred to as the funnest, craziest person to work with: a ball of energy. It helped my career because clients thought I was so funny and charming. No one was worried about me, and I would have laughed at them if they had been.

Over the next couple of years, I lived a jet-set lifestyle, moving between jobs in New York, London and Berlin. I was constantly jet-lagged, rarely sleeping on flights, with racing thoughts about possible business ventures, magazines I could maybe shoot for, and pictures I could take. Despite the lack of sleep, my energy levels were ridiculously high. On some days, I was even running half marathons with ease. Deep down, I knew it wasn't normal. I'd begun to lie to my mum on the phone, telling her I was tired from my busy days (when really, I felt the exact opposite).

Among these periods of hyperactivity were some days when I would completely crash and feel down and depressed. I was living in my manager's flat for a period of time and she was barely there, so I became comfortable with keeping my low moods a secret. They never lasted too long, so I just put it down to the swings and roundabouts of a model's lifestyle. Everyone gets sad sometimes, right?

By 2017, I was mostly back in Europe, due to fewer opportunities in New York and more in London. This was the year I met my then boyfriend – let's call him B – through a dating app. It was my first time falling in love (I quickly realised cool indie boy from school was an obsession, not love).

From the first date, I think we knew that it was more than something casual – we just couldn't get enough of each other. There was a magnetic pull between us that I had never felt before. Introducing each other to our families felt so natural. We slotted into each other's lives effortlessly. He worked in the music industry, and we bonded over our ambition, loving supporting each other in our careers. We were both social creatures, so we quickly became equally enmeshed in each other's social lives.

We did everything together: dinner parties, festivals, lazy Sunday mornings and walks to get coffee. It just felt so easy. We didn't really argue, and I felt that I could rely on him. I never felt lonely when we were together. I split my time between my parents' house in Edgware Road and B's flat in South West London, working non-stop for high-profile brands such as ASOS, while keeping up running and going to yoga classes. I finally felt comfortable in my own skin and started to enjoy experimenting with my outfit choices (I had a penchant for fun, colourful trainers). I was living the kind of life that I had dreamed of for my early twenties. I was thriving, or so I thought. Little did I know that life would soon come crashing down.

2
going south

I started 2018 in a pretty normal way for a twenty-two year old: at a house party taking MDMA (ecstasy). I remember feeling like I LOVED LIFE, telling all my friends how much they meant to me. (Later, I would panic that this drug was the trigger that changed my brain chemistry forever, but I was reassured by doctors that it wasn't.) I fell asleep as the sun rose, excited about what the next year could bring to my already blissful life. I was especially excited for the holiday that B and I had booked to India – we were flying out there the next day. We had booked it months before. Feeling increasingly burned out from work, we both wanted some time together, just the two of us. B had planned a trip to Venice for my birthday a few months earlier, so it was my turn to do all the admin. I booked our flights and some beautiful accommodation. I couldn't wait for winter sun, romance and curry.

During this holiday, my high-energy bubble that had mostly lasted for the past few years abruptly burst. On our first stop in Mumbai, as we explored the flower markets,

I became overwhelmed by how busy it was (unusual for me) and increasingly irritable. I was constantly pushing for an argument with B. I remember going for dinner one night and bringing up my exes and past relationships almost solely to create drama, which understandably made B feel confused and defensive. It was very out of character, as we hardly ever argued. I felt so annoyed and unsettled and assumed the jet lag had thrown me off. After my bipolar diagnosis, I noticed that jet lag is a trigger for me – it sends me into either a high or a low. Now, I'm prescribed sleeping pills to ensure the impact of long-haul flights is minimal. On our last night in Mumbai, I curled up on the bed, repeating the fact that I felt overwhelmed. It wasn't a word I used very often and definitely didn't describe my usual character.

We went on to Goa, where we stayed in an idyllic hotel by the beach. There, my mood went from 0 to 100 when I saw how beautiful our room was. I felt so happy and so lucky that I immediately burst into tears. That night, I drank a lot of wine, and the next morning I was back to feeling 0 once more. I woke up at 8 a.m. (much later than my usual 5 a.m.), with no energy for my morning run. I wondered why I was so deeply overcome with sadness when I was in the most beautiful location with the person I loved.

I tried to suppress my feelings as I didn't want to ruin the holiday we'd been looking forward to for so long. But I couldn't deny that something was up. I had a horrible feeling in my stomach for the rest of the trip, as if something bad was about to happen. I started to worry about my life and what it would be like after the trip, and I began to overexercise again. I kept thinking that my success as a model had been a fluke – that I wasn't pretty enough to keep it going. Then what would I do? B was so confused – this wasn't the excitable, happy Rosie he knew. While I was calling my mum multiple times a day in need of reassurance, he lay on the beach, wondering who the hell I was and what I had done with his fun-loving girlfriend.

Arriving back in the UK, I had three weeks of work lined up, but this stifling feeling that my career was spiralling downwards continued. Having my make-up and hair done at work, I started feeling like a fraud, paranoid that everyone on set was questioning why I was getting so much work.

One day, I was working at a photo shoot for a well-known brand. The building we were in was undergoing construction works when I suddenly felt the ground drop beneath my feet. I quickly sat down. My heart was racing and I started to shake. I asked everyone in the room if they had felt the drop too, jumping up with an urgent feeling of needing to leave the building in case we were unsafe. Another model on set could see that I was distressed and comforted me. She said she hadn't felt anything and everyone else agreed. Despite her reassurance, I couldn't get my heart to slow down; I felt dizzy and sick. I left work early, which made me feel embarrassed and even more convinced that my days as a model were over.

My mum was away at the time, as was B, so the only reassurance came from telling myself that it was probably just an ear infection. I lay down for the rest of the day and booked to see a doctor the next morning. There, I recited the symptoms of an ear infection I had read about online rather than being completely honest about my increasing anxiety. All I wanted was for them to tell me my ears were infected and send me away with antibiotics.

This turned out to be the first of six doctors' appointments over the next two weeks. Every time I got up to walk around, I felt the ground dropping again and the sickness continued. I ran the course of antibiotics yet felt no improvement, so I kept booking in to see different doctors. I was beginning to develop completely irrational thoughts that I was about to die, and that nobody had found the *real* reason for my illness. I grew even more anxious and was becoming increasingly exhausted, but still couldn't sleep.

On a Sunday evening, after a week of being in bed and incessantly Googling my symptoms, I called my mum in crisis. My heart was beating so fast this time that I screamed down the phone to her that I was dying – that the sensations in my body were unbearable. And so, that night, I found myself in A&E, hoping that doctors would now take my health seriously and do some kind of heart scan.

This was my first experience of a panic attack. My sister Lucy heard what had happened and came to my side. We sat in the waiting room before a doctor looked at my ears again and checked my heart, before suggesting that anxiety was the real cause of what was going on after weeks of complete confusion. I couldn't believe it, and even doubted his opinion. I couldn't get my head around the idea that anxiety could cause such intense physical symptoms.

I was diagnosed with panic disorder and generalised anxiety disorder, and started the process of trying several different antidepressant medicines, none of which seemed to stick. I couldn't think further than a day ahead; I was just focused on remembering how to breathe around others. I became incredibly disengaged, where I just wanted to make it to the end of the day without having a panic attack. I was stunned by how severe panic attacks were, and I found myself feeling angry, upset and irritable. I couldn't wrap my head around such a difficult existence after years of feeling on top of the world.

The most worrying symptom of the anxiety was hearing voices in my head. I knew everyone had an internal monologue that could get louder in difficult times, but I tried to explain to my mum and B that the volume of the voices wasn't normal. I would have to listen to rap music or walk near roadworks just to block out their intensity.

The voices were at their worst whenever I was at work; it felt as if someone was constantly shouting at me, telling me I wasn't good enough for the job. *You're ugly. You're lazy. These brands don't want you here – you're a disappointment.* It felt as if I was being bullied.

On a shoot, a stylist opened up to me, telling me how 'life had never felt the same again' when she developed anxiety. I stopped replying to her messages after that, and distanced myself, because at that time I needed reassurance. It upset me so much hearing those words that I began to sink into depression, believing this was my life from now on. To this day, I struggle being around people who make me believe I'll never get better.

I was barely seeing friends, and my withdrawal from social situations began to affect my relationship. Every night I saw B, I would cry. I was upset if he wanted to go to parties or events without me, but insisted I couldn't go with him. I was irritable, insecure and angry at the situation, as I festered on how he could 'choose' to do other things rather than stay in with me. Depression really brings out the diva!

If you've struggled with mental illness, you'll know that in these low moments, the mind loves to tell you that *nobody* has ever felt like this – that you are alone, that you're broken. Of course, that's not rational, but when you're in the thick of it, you have blinkers on and can't necessarily access those rational thoughts. Even when you know other people struggle too (such as the girl I met on the shoot), the voice in your head can be so confident in isolating you and preventing you from finding comfort in other people's experiences.

I skipped between medicines – none of them were changing my thoughts and, if anything, I was getting worse. Looking back now, I can see where my bipolar was so obvious. I'd even written in my diary every week or two about these fleeting 'positive days' when I had so much energy and felt I was getting better – which I now know were signals of hypomania. When you're in a bad place and you have a good day, you don't see that as a warning sign. You think of it as a relief.

Around three weeks after starting a new medicine, I was at dinner with my friend Sophia. My head started to hurt – it felt like everything inside it was rejigging itself. There was a rush of adrenaline as my mind told me that an antidepressant was finally working – maybe the end was in sight! I bounced home for the first time in months not feeling anxious.

I called B when I got home. 'B, I can't explain it, but I'm feeling so much better – I think the medication is working!' I exclaimed.

'Bloody hell, Rosie, that's a relief,' he replied. 'You sound better.'

'I *am* better! I think my brain chemistry has shifted. Let's do something nice tomorrow – I want to see you,' I said. 'I know everything has been shit lately, but I think it's going to be better now.'

'That's amazing, Rosie. Thank fuck the medication is finally working,' he replied, before we decided to meet at Kew Gardens.

The next day, I turned up at Kew to meet him, beaming. I hadn't slept and my headaches had continued. Despite this,

I didn't feel anxious at all. My mind was racing with endless positive thoughts and grand ideas about what I would do with my life in good health. B commented on how beautiful I looked, and I remember thinking that everyone in the park thought the same. I was in my prime: an obvious model to anyone walking past. We laughed the whole morning. My brain was going off in random tangents, darting all over the place, which made me funnier than ever. It felt so effortless and easy between us, just as it had been when we first got together.

At the café, I ordered us two slices of cake. As we ate, I thought to myself, *This is what I'm going to do every Saturday afternoon, now I've got this new-found joy about life again.* I texted my mum telling her that citalopram had 'cured my anxiety and depression'. I was tearful with the belief that I could be waking up from the horrible nightmare I'd been living in.

I texted all my friends to meet at the pub that evening to celebrate this news, all the while with manic thoughts racing through my brain. (I'll put these manic thoughts in capitals throughout the book as I'm sure anyone who has experienced them will know it's a pretty loud internal voice!)

> I'M SO IN LOVE.
> I'M SO HAPPY.
> I'M FREE FROM ANXIETY.
> I CAN'T WAIT TO DRINK A COCKTAIL.
> I CAN'T WAIT TO SOCIALISE AGAIN.

Later that evening, sitting at the pub, cocktail in hand, I was talking more in an hour than I potentially had in three months. All I wanted to do was explain how *happy* I was. I couldn't stop saying it, welling up and laughing.

Nobody could understand the leap I had taken to get here. At one point, B cut in with, 'Rosie, you used to be happy. You never used to have to say it.'

The comment threw me. It made me feel deeply embarrassed, and I suddenly became aware of just how much I had been speaking. I was offended by him putting me down.

'You just don't understand how ill I've been,' I snapped at him.

We left the pub soon after, and I woke up the next day feeling just as depressed as I had before.

As the summer months started to creep up, I began to feel worse than ever. Even the beautiful weather couldn't lift my mood. I felt numb, exhausted and disinterested. Ironically, my career was going better than ever – my anxiety-induced weight loss went down a hit at work for all the wrong reasons, and I felt that I couldn't say no to jobs when I was earning so much every week.

One day, I received an email from my agency while I was on a shoot, telling me I would have to fly to Italy for a job the next day. Then the make-up artist told me I needed to pluck my eyebrows and my skin wasn't good, which spun me out. Having modelled for years by this point, I was used to these comments and could normally handle them. But I suddenly felt extremely sensitive and hated that people were touching my face and hair. This brought on an immediate panic attack in front of the team I was working with. I was hyperventilating and could barely get my words out. The photographer was kind and understanding and suggested I take a walk at lunch. I ran out of the studio and sat down at a busy roundabout and called my mum.

'I feel like I'm falling apart,' I told her, tears bursting from my eyes, as she tried to soothe me and remind me to breathe.

Eventually, I calmed down enough to return to the studio, feeling hopeful that I could get on with my job.

As soon as I walked back in, the make-up artist scolded me for ruining my eye make-up. In that moment, I realised I just couldn't do it anymore. I couldn't keep acting as if I was fine. I was clearly in crisis.

For the first time that year, I called my agency to tell them I was struggling severely with my mental health and needed to leave work. Thankfully, they were understanding and allowed me to take some time off. One of my bookers had a daughter who struggled with mental illness, so she said she understood and reassured me that it was okay to get help and no one would think badly of me, given I had always been so reliable. I sat outside, cradling myself, embarrassed, while my mum drove across London to collect me.

I spent four days at home with my parents in Edgware Road in a crisis, thinking that if I wasn't modelling, I wouldn't know how to spend my days. I had to cancel jobs that had already been confirmed, which I had never done before. Everyone knew me as the busiest model, so stopping work to get help felt like the biggest obstacle. My mind told me I was pathetic, the agency hated me and nobody believed I was ill (despite my booker telling me otherwise). After a week, I felt so annoyed at myself for not being able to hold it together that I went back to work without addressing the issue. I thought that if I could just push through, things would start to improve.

It was during this time that I first heard the word 'bipolar' uttered by a new GP on a visit about changing my medication, accompanied by my mum. He was the first person to ask me whether I have positive days among the awful ones. When I said I sometimes experienced bursts of energy, he tentatively asked, 'Have you considered the possibility of bipolar disorder?'

My mum responded immediately with anger. 'How dare you suggest something like that,' she retorted. She resented the implication that he was trying to paint me as 'crazy' or 'mad', rather than a normal young adult suffering from anxiety and depression in an unstable phase of life.

I didn't really know much about bipolar at the time – I probably would have described the weather as bipolar on one of those weird sunny-then-rainy-then-sunny-again days. But I took on my mum's anger; it felt as if the doctor was accusing me of something, rather than helping me. I felt a panic attack rising in my chest.

'Come on, Rosie, we're leaving,' my mum said, and we stormed out of the room – without even giving the GP the chance to respond.

We went back to my parents' office, where my dad was equally outraged to hear the doctor's comment. My parents then spoke to friends who work in the medical field; they agreed that it was unprofessional for a GP to mention a label like that to me at a first meeting when they're not allowed to diagnose.

Looking back, my mum doesn't regret her reaction. She just wanted to protect me, and I think a lot of people have these moments of denial when they're first confronted with the reality of their mental health. Saying this, I do sometimes think about what might have been different if I'd listened and pursued a diagnosis at that time. Maybe I would have received the help I needed sooner. Maybe I would have avoided sinking into psychosis.

* * *

Life went on, despite having panic attacks and crying every evening. My relationship broke down; I had become a shadow of the person B first met. I knew, deep down, that it was over. My mental health had become the only thing I could speak about, and I felt like a burden to everyone around me – especially him.

On the last day of August, I met B in Primrose Hill, knowing an honest conversation was finally about to happen after months of not communicating properly. I remember trying to laugh while I was crying, and blurting out, 'I can't believe you're going to fucking dump me.' I refused to look him in the eye until we sat down on the grass.

'Rosie, I've felt like this for a long time now,' B said. 'I'm sure it's the right thing.' He promised me he'd only mentioned it to his mum. He was going to LA in a few months' time, and he explained that he needed to concentrate on work.

He said the words, but I wasn't really focusing. I was trying to imagine what my life would be after this break-up. B felt like the only thing I had left. How would I survive without him? What the McShit would I do when the only person I spoke to wasn't there for me anymore?

As I flitted between laughing and crying, I heard myself say, 'I love you so much' to him.

He didn't say it back.

The voice in my head started having a field day. *Rosie, you're absolutely pathetic.* Suddenly, I could see the funny side. How had I become this insecure person, desperately trying to get a boy to like me when clearly it wasn't working? It felt like a reality check.

When there were no tears left to cry, I felt a bizarre sense of relief. I thought it could be quite funny to make him feel even worse if I acted really unhinged. Given my mental state for the last eight months, I thought, *Might as well shove the dagger in and make him think this will make everything even worse.*

I insisted he leave, telling him I was going to sit on the top of the hill by myself, 'and maybe get a drink,' hinting that I planned to get drunk on my own.

'Rosie – please go and be with some friends,' B insisted.

'Nope. I'm fine, thank you. Please leave me alone,' I retorted, before saying, 'I want to be alone all night. I don't know what is going to happen…'

I knew full well this would make him worry, and for some reason I took pride in that. Eventually, he agreed to leave. As soon as he was out of sight, I walked home, texting my sisters with two simple instructions: 1) come round ASAP, and 2) bring prosecco. We ended up laughing all evening, and I felt the best I had for weeks. I assumed it was just because my ex had been weighing me down, and now I was 'cured'.

B and I had a short getaway to Amsterdam booked for that weekend, and my oldest sister Amii kindly agreed to drop her plans to come with me so I wouldn't have to cancel it. The day we arrived, I was so anxious that we spent the entire day looking for a pharmacy to find some anti-anxiety medicines. We ate dinner in the hotel because I was too scared to go out. But the next day, I had done a full 180 (you'll notice this happens a lot…).

'I'm going to meet my Dutch friend Evelyn for drinks,' I told my sister, not even considering how rude it was to ditch her on a holiday for just the two of us.

Evelyn arrived at my hotel to find me in the shadow of a champagne bottle. I soon became quick-witted, funny and very, very drunk.

Long story short, I ended up fainting in a very cool rooftop bar (twice) and throwing up (far more than that). At 1 a.m., I was crying to my sister in our hotel bedroom (while trying to stomach a chocolate bar). I felt a sense of disassociation from what had just happened and couldn't explain my behaviour. I told her I got carried away with the champagne, but in all honesty it felt as though my apology was on behalf of someone else. Someone I couldn't relate to.

My sister called my mum to explain what had happened, and the word 'bipolar' was brought up again. Weeks earlier, Amii had been the only one who wasn't shocked by the suggestion when my parents relayed what the GP had said.

'Do you think it could be bipolar?' I heard her ask them over the phone. 'Rosie *is* so up and down.'

My parents listened to her but disagreed, telling her that at my age I was just going through a bad time and it was never going to last.

Amii handed the phone over to me.

'You need a proper break, Rose,' my mum said. She was in Croatia on holiday with my dad, Lucy and her boyfriend. 'Can you let your agency know that you're coming out to join us here for a few days? What about at the end of next week?'

The voice of authority had spoken; my mum's tone was firm. Cuddles and some sunshine sounded great. My flight was booked for just over a week's time, but I wouldn't end up boarding the plane.

3
unravelling

I find this part of that whole sorry year to be the most difficult to recount. In just under a fortnight between my chaotic Amsterdam trip and my flight to Croatia, I would spiral into a psychosis so severe that it would take months (in fact, years) to recover.

I returned from Amsterdam to an Indian summer in London. Weirdly, September has always been my favourite month. It still feels like the start of school and, maybe because of working in fashion, it has always felt more like the new year than January has. It's typically the time when I feel most contemplative. Breaking up with my boyfriend and having glorious weather and a holiday booked with my family felt very surreal and exciting.

Arriving back in London, I decided it was time to get moving on my post-break-up glow. The next day, I woke up early. Instead of being filled with anxious thoughts, I walked to a yoga class feeling Zen. *Why am I not anxious?* I thought to myself. *What has changed? Am I cured? This definitely doesn't feel like depression!*

I swanned into the class, very confident, speaking openly to the teacher beforehand about my recent break-up and my plans to do yoga every single morning for seven days. During the flow, I felt unusually present and connected to my body. Then, in the meditative section of the class, I reached a feeling of complete stillness. Of course, so many people love yoga for this exact reason, but it wasn't something I was usually able to achieve – my mind was normally so busy and active. Yet this time I felt a profound sense of peace. It was invigorating.

After the class, as I looked at myself in the changing-room mirrors, I was met by extremely kind, but intense, thoughts on my appearance. During the past year, I had felt rock bottom about my appearance and questioned my longevity as a model, but now I was full of adoration for how I looked.

> YOU'VE GOT AMAZING SKIN!
> YOU'RE GLOWING! THIS IS A NEW LIFE!
> YOU'RE SO YOUNG!
> YOU HAVE EVERYTHING AHEAD OF YOU!

I wasn't used to this, but my God, I wasn't going to complain. As I stared in the mirror, I began to see myself as an old woman. I didn't question this strange vision – instead, I believed I had unlocked this superpower. I could see the future and knew how my destiny was going to play out for me. I snapped a selfie and posted it on Instagram, calling myself a 'North London mum' in my tight leggings and oversized hoodie, repeatedly refreshing the page to see who had reacted. I was quite sure that the boys who followed me would think I looked fantastic and that my next boyfriend was imminent.

By the time I reached work, I had sent multiple texts to people I knew I needed to see ASAP.

Hey Alice! I'm back from work late on Wednesday ... wanna do a night out? Really need one after my break-up lol x

Hi Luce! Are you around this week? I'm joining the rents next week but would love to see you before I go :) Shall I come and collect you from work on Thursday? And we can have a drink?

Creates group WhatsApp

Hey guys! Really want to do a roast on Sunday – fancy meeting at The Spaniards at around 13.00? I'm going to do yoga in the morning first if anyone wants to join me

Hi mummy – I'm SO excited for our holiday!! Thank you so much for organising!! I've texted Christine to do my last session of therapy the night before I come out ... I can't explain it but I think I'm cured?! Will call later xxx

My excitement for life skyrocketed. In the days that followed, I was barely sleeping, managing little more than two hours a night. My head was full of business ideas and things I *needed* to write down. Listening to rap music, I believed the lyrics were about *my* life. I texted my friends telling them how much I loved them, bought a designer bag, went out drinking every evening, and started over-exercising again, going for runs twice a day.

I'd grown up as an atheist – one of my earliest memories was my mum telling me that God didn't exist, a belief she'd had since losing her young son to cancer. But suddenly I felt profoundly spiritual. God *had* to be involved with the way I was feeling. I had never felt more sure of anything in my life. I felt the opposite of alone; I felt empowered and seen. The weirdest aspect of delusion is how quickly it becomes normalised, and how you simply don't judge how different your beliefs are from weeks earlier.

> GOD IS DOING THIS.
> YOUR LIFE IS ABOUT TO CHANGE.
> YOU ARE THE CHOSEN ONE.
> EVERYTHING IS HAPPENING FOR A REASON.
> YOU HAVE ONLY BEEN ILL SO YOU CAN NOW ENJOY GOOD HEALTH.
> EVERYONE LOVES YOU.
> YOU ARE SO TALENTED.
> YOU ARE THE WORLD'S BEST MODEL.
> YOU HAVE SO MUCH TO GIVE!
> HAVE ANOTHER BEER!
> CELEBRATE!

Looking back, I now understand that grand spiritual thoughts are a key warning sign for psychosis. But I just felt that I was having sparkling moments of realisation, and I'd never felt so good. I started sharing some of my profound thoughts on my social media, leading one of my friends to message me: *You sound manic, Rosie, are you okay?* I was absolutely furious and responded by continuing to share even more spiritual stories, including one where I outed their comment online, expressing my rage at that judgement.

I continued sharing long essays online about how I had learnt to love myself and found balance. My hunger felt bottomless – I was eating about seven meals a day – and yet my clothes seemed to be falling off me.

In one selfie I shared on Instagram, I noticed how slim I was looking after a few days of running around with crazy energy. Like everything that week, I felt the world was waiting on every thought of mine, leading me to share the picture along with the caption: *I don't know what is happening to me but my metabolism feels like a seven-year-old boy's.*

As I hit share, I had an epiphany that maybe I didn't just feel like a seven-year-old boy, but there was a greater spiritual cause as well. Texting my mum in a manic tone, I asked her to confirm at what age my brother had died from leukaemia. *I must be a reincarnation of Alex*, I thought. Tears poured down my cheeks as I stopped to think what this meant. I had always known something was different about me – was this it? Was I Alex coming back to life? Perhaps this is what was causing my new-found lust for life?

Weirdly, this epiphany came about on set when I was surrounded by a whole team of people. I was talking a million miles an hour, shaking and asking the make-up artist if she would drink prosecco on the train ride home with me. Oddly, no one followed up to check whether I was okay. No one rang my modelling agent. No one could put a finger on what I was experiencing. Maybe they all just believed I was on drugs.

The night before I was due to fly out to Croatia, I sat at the bar of a pub near my house. I was waiting for my 'last' therapy session, unbelievably excited to explain the epiphanies I had recently had. It was weird to see the street in a different headspace. Usually, I would make sure that the journey from the station to the therapy door was as quick as possible, taking the bus and drowning out my thoughts with loud music. This time, I arrived two hours early and walked from the station to the pub with the sun on my face, listening to the sounds of the world, excited to write in my diary and refuel (potentially my fifth meal that day). I ordered beef ragu pasta and whizzed through two glasses of prosecco, chatting to the bartender about my love of life while writing.

In my therapy session, I wittered away about my grand ideas and spiritual awakening, but my therapist didn't pick up on anything being amiss. She just thought I had turned a corner. When I reflect on this now, I feel resentful that she didn't pick up on the signs of bipolar and that I was heading into a dangerously manic episode. But at the same time, I do wonder, would I have even listened if she had?

Climbing into bed that night, having posted about twenty times that day on social media, I looked down at my phone and suddenly felt a wave of panic. I deleted everything I had shared that day on my stories, removed the app, and embraced the holiday mindset of being off-grid. Something deep down inside me knew that what I had shared hadn't been normal. I suddenly wanted to be with my mum and started to feel agitated that my friends hadn't responded to any of my stories beyond concerned texts and missed calls. *Why was everyone being so negative?*

***

At 4 a.m. the next day, I woke up and bounced out of bed. My hands were shaking as adrenaline pumped around my body. The original plan for that day was breakfast with a friend in a café in Angel (in London) at 9 a.m., then on to catch my flight at 3 p.m. from Stansted Airport. I couldn't understand why I was so hungry and restless. Without questioning too much, I grabbed two bananas from the kitchen, devoured them quickly, and set off a few minutes later for a long run. My breathing was heavy and my mind was in a trance as I sprinted around the park. Tears began to stream from my eyes. It was an uncomfortable anticipation, but I knew ... *I was about to meet God.*

The tears kept coming. I was experiencing a natural ecstasy. As I got closer to my house, I was suddenly struck with an unbearable hunger again. A man sitting outside a shisha bar noticed my tearful face and fidgety mannerisms and insisted I sit down next to him and drink some water. My perception of time from this point onwards went completely out the window. It wasn't until 9.30 a.m., when I received a worried message from my friend, sitting alone at our breakfast date, that I realised how much time had passed.

You okay?!! she sent, with a photo of an empty café.

One moment, the world was whizzing by all around me, and the next it felt like I was existing in slow motion. I was no longer experiencing time at a consistent rate: psychosis had a full grip on me. What I do remember is sitting in the shisha bar, enjoying a huge plate of biscuits that had kindly been offered to me. I turned to my phone, looking up the route to get to Angel on Citymapper. However, instead of showing me a bus route, my app seemed to delete every icon – and a spaceman suddenly appeared, hinting that I could teleport there if I wanted to. I remember laughing, thinking this was God's banter, before watching the app plan out a single bus route I could take.

Psychosis was the most surreal experience I have ever had – and I can't even claim that it was all terrible. At points, it felt like taking the strongest stimulant possible; the kind of experience a lot of people would pay good money for. Every single thing that happens feels as though it is supposed to.

I got on a bus and headed to Baker Street. Hopping off as quickly as I had boarded it, I felt an intense feeling of restlessness. The location of King's Cross suddenly felt important. I ran and ran and ran, eventually reaching the main entrance to the station.

Then, another moment of awe overcame me. This time, I found myself in McDonald's. Starving, and already imagining the delicious taste of cheeseburger in my mouth, I dashed for the entrance. I took the orders of two homeless men who were sitting outside, before marching to the front and looking lovingly at the woman serving me. She was so beautiful. I paused to think about why our paths had crossed and what this moment meant. Fidgeting and talking to everyone else waiting, I grabbed the order and delivered the porridge pots to the men outside. They thanked me for being 'a hero'

YOU HAVEN'T SEEN ANYTHING YET,
I thought, while rushing off with a quick 'God bless you'.
I AM HERE TO SAVE THE WORLD.
I WILL DO ALL I CAN TO MAKE SURE PEOPLE ARE HAPPY.
WHERE IS GOD?!
IS HE HERE?!
MAYBE HE'S IN ANGEL?!

I ran up the steep hill from King's Cross to Angel, darting in front of cars, causing several to honk at me. I stopped to steal a lemon from M&S, biting into it in the street while looking for a coffee shop. Caffeine was like rocket fuel, and I craved it. Entering one coffee shop nearby, I was suddenly struck with a wave of sadness and a sudden fear that I didn't know what was happening. I burst into tears, and the owner comforted me as I let out a scream. I was distressed, heavily emotional and in crisis.

WHY IS GOD NOT HERE?!
WHERE IS MY MUM?!
WHO IS THIS MAN?!

I spotted that the café had a second floor. I wanted peace and quiet so went upstairs and hid, cradling my head with my hands in frustration. The voices no longer sounded warm and reassuring. They sounded menacing. When the owner turned his back, I rushed towards the spiralled stairway. The top floor had a prominent open window, and my mind told me to jump.

I get emotional when I think about this moment because I truly believed God would have saved me that day. I believed I was invincible, and it was incredibly dangerous. Fortunately, a customer grabbed my arm and pulled me into his chest. I was in trouble now – there was no way this behaviour could be deemed as normal. The owner sat and monitored me while discussing with the customers what best to do.

'Is she on drugs?'
'Can someone call the police?'
'Do we call an ambulance?'

I ran away when I found a suitable opportunity, fuelled by pure adrenaline. I still think about the kindness of the stranger who saved me from jumping. I also feel a deep sadness that I was alone, running around in complete confusion with no grasp on reality.

When I saw another coffee shop, I wanted to admit defeat. Then, another text came in from my friend who

I was supposed to meet: *Where are you?!* My perception of time returned – something I hadn't had a grip on for some time – and I realised that God hadn't come to find me yet.

By this point, I was mentally exhausted. Thanks to the many coffees I'd fuelled myself with, I was shaking and acutely aware of my loud heartbeat. I walked into the coffee shop and went up to the server, asking for a gingerbread latte, caramel biscuit and pack of peppermint chewing gum (three things I typically hate). As I sat down, I sipped a coffee that someone had left on the table in front of me (definitely my usual order), before putting my head between my legs.

I began to cry hysterically, and a man came to sit down opposite me. He introduced himself as Bill. Unaware of my morning, he simply smiled, trying to lift me from my tears. He was glowing (no exaggeration), and I felt my negative thoughts transform into positive ones once more. A sense of calm came over me. I felt comforted by this beautiful man who was curious to figure out who I was and why I was crying on the other side of his breakfast.

Chewing on my biscuit, which felt like I was eating cardboard, I noticed Bill had ordered my favourite breakfast: porridge and orange juice. I stared longingly at it. Seeing the envy in my eyes, he pushed the bowl towards me. It felt like a peace offering: a kind gift for his new tearful friend. His kindness lifted me out of my fearful headspace, and my godly thoughts returned. I feverishly explained to him that we were supposed to meet that morning. I believed God had led me through the day, and the penny dropped that he'd guided me to this moment. *Blond, glowy Bill must be the love of my life!*

THIS IS GOD'S PLAN!

We spoke about classical music, our love for our families and God knows what else. I don't know how long we were speaking; it felt like days but it may have only been a few minutes. I felt myself instantly fall in love. I was safe again and sure that we would be joined at the hip from here on out. Sadly, with Bill having to go to work, and me needing to pack for Croatia, we left the coffee shop to return to our respective days, albeit besotted with one another.

I felt the words, 'Will you marry me?' coming up my throat and blurted them out as he was putting his jacket on. Laughing at my 'sense of humour', he smiled and walked with me out of the coffee shop. We exchanged numbers, before kissing under the bus stop outside. It seemed sort of wild that this man thought I was some kind of manic pixie dream girl and not, you know, actually manic.

Bill left to catch the train to work, while I stood on the street and began calling and texting my friends, including one very questionable message to my ex.

Hey B!! I just wanted to say that I hope you find love again. You deserve to be with Ariana Grande SO much … I just want to see you happy!! I met the love of my life in a coffee shop this AM, LOL. Life is weird but sending lots of love!! Rosie xx

Hey R, I'm so sorry I missed breakfast. My phone died and I have had the weirdest morning! I will explain once back from holiday and breakfast is definitely on me!

Hi mumma. Call me ASAP!! I've met the love of my life in a coffee shop!

Calls modelling agency

'Hey! It's Rosie! Please can I speak to T? … AHHHHHH you'll never guess WHAT! I just met the love of my life in a coffee shop! He loves classical music too! I can't wait to come back to work after my holiday! Can we meet ASAP as I'd also love to talk to you guys about some campaigns I want to do? GREAT. SPEAK SOON!'

After all of this, I lay face down in an Uber and headed home to pack my bag.

I called Bill, who was walking from the station to his office. 'I think we should move in together.'

Clearly, he just thought I was being enthusiastic. He laughed and asked me questions about my life. It must have only been a five-minute conversation, but I felt as if we were connecting on the deepest level imaginable. He told me that he was buying his own flat and planned to set up a company with his brother. I told him about my family and friends and that I couldn't wait for him to meet them.

While he spoke, I imagined my whole life with him. I could picture myself walking down the aisle towards him and having children together. I rationalised that this must have been why my day had felt so weird. *It was all leading up to this magic, falling-in-love moment!*

On arriving home, I decided that I didn't really need to pack clothes – I could buy those. All I needed was my passport and a packet of All-Bran (an essential, of course), so I chucked them into a suitcase and zipped it up.

ROSIE. YOU'RE RUNNING LATE FOR YOUR FLIGHT.

I called another cab to take me to the airport, making sure the driver stopped off in Islington en route so I could grab a frozen yoghurt (with multiple toppings) for the journey. While I was spooning the yogurt into my mouth, the cab driver chatted away to me about his plans to create a rival to Uber with a fairer rate for the drivers. I kept feeling that I needed to help everyone I met, so I took his details and promised him that when I became a millionaire, I would get in touch to fund the initiative.

Eventually, the driver dropped me off outside the entrance to the airport terminal. As I jumped out of the car, my head began to hurt. There was just so much detail around me. As I stepped through the entrance, I lost all sense of how airports operate – I was overwhelmed by all the signs and the people, and I wasn't sure what it all meant. I asked a few strangers where I could find the luggage drop-off. Directed to a long queue, I stood still and cushioned my (basically empty) suitcase between my legs.

If you have ever experienced psychosis, you won't second-guess me when I tell you that time morphed into a different pace. As before, I began to feel as if I was existing in slow motion. Simply turning my head felt like a huge gesture. Tears began to stream from my eyes as I struggled to get my head around what was happening. I knew I needed help.

Finding my phone, I called my mum. 'Mummy,' I cried. 'I don't know what's happening – I can't get on this flight.'

'Rosie, this flight was expensive!' my mum snapped in response, frustrated that I didn't seem to be making any sense. 'You can't stay in London just because of this new man! Please get yourself checked-in!'

I dropped the phone, abandoned my bags and started running around the airport, again looking for signs from God about what to do. I didn't know the answer, and the voices in my head were confusing and frightening.

GO BACK TO LONDON, one prominent voice told me as I ran towards the train station. *GOD IS AROUND THE CORNER, ROSIE.*

I asked a man if he knew where God was, and if I could have his train ticket.

'Leave me alone,' he shouted. 'Of course you can't have my ticket.'

I was scared and confused. Why was nothing I tried leading me to clarity? I was constantly moving between reality and unreality. Nothing was in order.

GO BACK AND GET THE FLIGHT.
HOLIDAY WILL BE AMAZING.
YOU ARE LATE AND YOU WILL MISS THIS.
JUST GET THE FLIGHT.

I looked back towards the bag drop, completely forgetting where I was supposed to be going and who I was even flying with. Staring up at the confusing and huge information board, I decided to go to a British Airways desk to ask for help.

The woman behind the desk asked me where I was going.

I couldn't remember so asked her which flights were leaving, hoping to jog my memory.

'We have New York? We have Iceland? Will you show me your passport and I can help you find your flight?'

I burst into tears again as the woman's face didn't match her voice – it sounded distorted and confusing. After running for the bathroom, I shut myself in a loo cubicle and screamed my name three times loudly. (This was definitely inspired by *Call Me By Your Name*, a film I had watched the previous week.) Nobody replied – the room just went silent, so I ran out again.

Coming out of the loos, I saw Bill – the love of my life! I ran over to him and kissed him. But it turned out he wasn't in fact Bill; it was actually a random man who was standing next to his girlfriend.

The woman, understandably, became very vocal about the incident: 'Who the hell are you?!' Her shouting made my reality seem like a nightmare.

I ran away again. I had no idea where I had left my bags. My dissociation continued. I no longer remembered why I was in an airport and ran in one direction, paranoid that I was being chased by the devil. I wanted to hide from the world and bury myself in shame. And that's when I spotted the oversized baggage drop-off.

A member of airport staff was standing next to a big curtain where a queue of people were placing their bags ready for the flights. My heart was going at a million miles an hour, and I knew I needed help. On the one hand, I wanted to find God behind those curtains, while on the other hand the scared child in me knew that I needed to get attention by creating the biggest scene possible.

I ran to the front of the queue and dived through the curtain flaps. I started crawling through all the bags and made eye contact with a security guard, who was clearly confused about what I was doing. I was aware that I was in big trouble. I looked around wildly, searching for something, anything to take me out of this chaos. My focus landed on a big red fire alarm on my left, and I set it off.

In that moment, I realised my actions would have consequences – and that God wasn't coming to save me. The sound of the alarms echoing through the airport would soon be replaced by the sound of an ambulance coming to take me away.

4
detached from reality

There I was, well and truly in the grip of severe psychosis. This manic high would last for the best part of three months, during which time I lived in a locked psychiatric ward. What happened there is a blur. I moved between hallucinations, moments of calm and moments of chaos. When you emerge from mania, it can be difficult to distinguish between what really happened and what was just a figment of your imagination. What I share here is a mixture of memories I have pieced together, along with insights that my family have told me in the years since then.

After setting off the fire alarm in Stansted Airport, I was taken to a small room with a few police officers. They soon realised that I was not in my right mind, given that I was talking nonsense and abruptly switched from appearing heavily distressed to finding everything extremely funny. Instead of pressing criminal charges, the officers called an ambulance. While we waited, I showed them my tattoos and rattled on about my future plans to go on holiday, marry Bill and finally find God. I remember a few of them trying not to laugh, and I am pretty sure that I called one woman 'Police Queen' and another man 'Policey McPolice'.

They asked me to sit up on a table. I was fidgety and dangled my legs, swaying back and forth in an attempt to break the tense atmosphere. I asked to see their tattoos and keenly observed them. When you are manic, you really see the beauty in people, their authenticity, and in that moment I couldn't have been more thrilled to be surrounded by a room of warm faces. I hadn't really registered that the scene in front of me was a result of the alarm incident moments earlier.

When the ambulance arrived, two of the police officers escorted me out of the room and through the airport. As they held onto both of my arms, the crowds seemed to part like the Red Sea to let us through. It all felt very biblical – *this must be part of God's plan!*

I was still getting higher and higher. Little did I know that the delusional thoughts had only really just begun. While climbing into the ambulance, I became aware of people staring at me. I pushed back against the police officers, as the ambulance workers took control from them and were quite firm with me. These small moments reminded me that my day had been anything but normal. My *behaviour* was anything but normal. Glimmers of reality cut through the mayhem in my mind, but these moments were always brief. Soon enough, I was successfully in the back of the ambulance, my mind running away with the fairies again.

A woman sat opposite me and asked a few questions while we drove to the nearest A&E. I can't recall what she looked like, but I know that she was warm and sweet, handing me water and holding my hand occasionally as we spoke over the muted sound of sirens.

'What is your name?'

'Rosie van Amerongen.' I felt excited when I spied my suitcase and bag in the corner. I was finally on my way to Croatia to meet my parents.

'Who would you like us to call for you?' she asked.

'Love of my life, please,' I responded. 'His name is Bill – his number is in my phone.'

I'm not exactly sure what happened when she called Bill, but I assume he explained that he didn't really know me and we'd only met that morning. I can just imagine his shock on hearing that the dream girl who had kissed him at a bus stop that morning was actually desperately in need of psychological help.

'Who else could we call?' she asked, after ending the call with him.

'Amii! My older sister!' I squealed. 'It would be great to speak to her actually. Maybe she can fly with me tomorrow on holiday instead?'

I felt completely normal as the woman asked more questions. She asked about my history with mental health, and I told her about my diagnoses of generalised anxiety disorder and panic disorder. I also told her that things had been really good since my break-up – that I had been feeling better than ever.

I played the role of a normal and fine person, maintaining eye contact while I calmly answered her questions. But in reality, I was completely delusional. I had barely registered that I was in an ambulance, and I didn't think to ask where we were going, or why we were going there. None of that seemed to matter. I was fixated on the idea of Bill and our morning kiss, and excited about the holiday I still believed I was going on. Although I could hear an ambulance siren, I couldn't seem to get a hold on reality, nor could I understand that this was all a result of how I was acting.

I arrived in A&E to a blur of faces in a waiting room. I smiled at everyone I passed. At some point, Amii showed up with her husband. She later told me that as soon as I saw her, I darted for the doors to try to run away. I don't recall the event. But reflecting on this now, I think it was likely that seeing someone I knew shattered the illusion that this was normal, that I was fine.

Every time the hospital staff tried to calm me down and take me back to my seat, I tried to escape. As a result, they put me in a room with a lockable door. The room was small, with a raised bed and a chair. Amii stayed with me, eventually getting me to calm down enough to cuddle her on the bed.

'I'm the reincarnation of Alex,' I kept telling her.

I was overcome with the mixed emotions that this epiphany sprung upon me; happiness that I was so connected to him, but also sadness that this had been hidden for my whole life. I felt so certain that this was true – as certain as knowing my own name.

Now, I get so upset thinking about how this must have felt for Amii, and all the traumatic memories that would have resurfaced for her, reminding her of the brother she lost when she was only a child herself. Here she was, back in hospital with a sibling – something she hoped would never happen again. I know my delusions about our brother were extremely scary and triggering for her, although she only told me that much later on. I wish I could erase a lot of the things I said and did in the peak of my mania, but this moment probably trumps all the rest.

I was barely aware of what was happening around me, but it turns out that we were waiting to find out if any beds had become available on mental health wards in nearby hospitals. In the meantime, my mum had booked the first possible late-night flight to land in London. By the morning, she had come to join us in A&E. My dad, in Croatia with their car, had a hero friend who offered to fly out to be with him on the long drive back to the UK. While I would love to tell you what it felt like to see my mum, who had flown back especially to be with me, I was stuck in slow motion with little awareness of what was unfolding. Instead, I was staring at the other patients and details of the hospital, which seemed enhanced by my superhuman eyesight.

While I was still in that small room, unable to sleep and swinging between intense joy and confusion, my mum called her friend Ian, a psychiatrist, to join us. She hoped he would be able to calm me down. His presence only served to confuse me more: for some reason, I thought he was my ex's dad, so I proceeded to tell him my side of the break-up as though he was a completely different person. Thankfully, he had plenty of experience with patients with psychosis so he was unfazed by my manic state. He stayed in the room with me throughout the night, his calm voice helping to soothe Amii and me. I remember the dimmed lights as she encouraged me to get some sleep, tightly holding onto me.

Although I didn't know Ian well, something about his tone felt safe. I am sure this is a result of years of work around manic people, but it was just what I needed to stop running away. I can't remember his appearance. I only remember his silhouette in the corridor, with lights shining through the door window behind his head.

Throughout the night, I was highly emotional – flitting between sadness and sheer panic as I realised my ex, B, wasn't nearby. Morning came, but I had barely slept. Ian and Amii had to get me to breathe slowly for hours on end. Apart from that feeling of safety from Ian, the only other thing I remember throughout that night was bursts of sadness and panic. These erupted into screams, and the trigger of the episode I was in began to come to the surface.

Not long after, my mum's sister Bella joined us. She ended up on the receiving end of my fatigue and poor humour. I laughed at her 'granny shoes' and ordered her to fetch me M&S sandwiches. By the second half of the night, my body had given up on me. My mind was getting more and more active, so when she came into the room all I remember was her gently patting me on my back while I stared at the floor beneath me.

After about 24 hours, we were told that a bed had become available. Mum and I sat in the back of another ambulance, which took us to Ealing Hospital in West London. (Apparently I told her that her shoes were hideous.)

My next memory is of being on the ward in Ealing Hospital, screaming for help, believing that the anti-psychotic injections which the nurses were pinning me down for to put into my bum were, in fact, cocaine. Quite a rock star explanation, I know, but reality was far away at this point. The lack of sleep meant my psychosis had worsened and paranoia had kicked in. The nurses became people from my past: their faces morphed, and their voices became distorted and loud. I was petrified. My reality felt like a nightmare.

Thanks to my screams and kicks, I was deemed a risk to the other patients and placed in seclusion for the first few days of my stay. Seclusion, which could also be called 'the worst place in the world', is a private room on a ward where nurses can look at you through a glass screen. During these days, my delusions were so strong that I spent most of my time crawling around on the floor with my eyes rolled back into my head.

My time in seclusion felt like a dystopian horror movie. There was a mattress in the left corner of the room.

I say 'mattress' loosely, because it was really just a huge plastic-covered pad. I am pretty sure it was exactly the same thing my school used on sports day when children attempted acrobatics for the first time and needed something big enough to land on. I don't recall anyone – no nurses or my mum – in the room with me. But I do remember Custard Cream and Bourbon deliveries through a hatch in the door.

With no natural light, the only way I could work out the time of day was by watching how many people were observing me from the other side of the glass. If there were several people, I assumed it was daytime. Sometimes, I would look up to see multiple smiling faces, giving me hope that I would soon be allowed to leave. In sadder moments, I was left with one man taunting me from the other side of the glass. He would put his thumbs in his ears and stick out his tongue, or he would raise his arms in the air and curl his hands into claws.

My mind had blocked out this memory until the week I left the hospital, when I spotted him in the hallway. I felt aggravated and upset, but I also knew that there was no point in filing a report on him. I was hardly a reliable witness, but I am adamant that this moment from my seclusion was real. It makes me feel unsafe and sad when I think about how vulnerable I was while in the grips of psychosis. If something really terrible had happened to me, I would never have been believed.

When you're experiencing an extreme manic episode, it can take several weeks for anti-psychotic medication to kick in. After a few days, I stopped kicking and screaming, but my delusions were still strong. I was soon moved to a standard bedroom, which was better than seclusion but still fairly basic. The room was designed to reduce the risk of patients harming themselves. There was a window in there, but it didn't open properly, and there were no curtains thanks to the suicide risk. There was no duvet cover – only one very thick sheet – and patients deemed to be high-risk weren't allowed in their rooms during the day. My mum brought a rug for the floor to make it feel more homely, and there was a red leathery chair that my parents would sit on when they visited. I had a sink, shelves and a tiny wardrobe that contained clothes folded neatly by my mum. I didn't wear most of them, mind you; I mainly lived in pyjamas. There weren't any mirrors anywhere (again, due to the suicide risk), so I couldn't have fussed over my appearance even if I had wanted to.

I was living on a women-only ward, which had room for around thirty women in total. It was housed on the seventh floor of the hospital behind a locked heavy-duty door. Sometimes, the patients would loiter next to it to try to escape (never with any luck ... at least not while I was there).

My room was one of twelve bedrooms at one end of the corridor. The main sitting room, containing three leather sofas and a TV, was across the hallway. There was a glass staff area, so we could be observed at all times. I had to ask permission to use the shower room, which I assume means I didn't shower at all in my first few weeks. I dread to think what I must have smelled like. Later during my stay, I discovered that patients (deemed low risk for suicide) could use a bath.

At this point during my psychosis, I believed I could pause time. While I splashed about having a great time, a nurse knocked on the door to say that my dad had arrived to visit me. I remember thinking, *I'm not finished yet*, and I clicked my fingers and paused the world while I continued to wash. The reality? My dad waited for forty-five minutes before having to leave because, obviously, my finger-clicking didn't quite work the way I wanted it to.

Then there was the medicine room, where we would line up after our meals to pick up our pills in tiny cardboard holders. I had no idea what these medicines were, but I remember knocking them back and being told I was good for doing so. It turns out that they were anti-psychotics, as well as tranquillisers, to keep me calmer around the nurses. On one manic day, I collected my medicines and threw them into a black bag as a cleaner walked past me. Generally though, I just did what I was told, as if I was back at school.

My favourite area was the dining room, where we would eat breakfast, lunch and dinner. My mania made everything taste incredible, and my appetite seemed to be bottomless. Mum later told me that she would bake cakes before her visits and I would happily devour an entire carrot cake or lemon loaf in one sitting, which she had hoped to share with the nurses looking after me. The meals we were served in hospital were just like the ones I had eaten in school, and I absolutely loved them. There were very few vegetables on offer; it was always a curry, lasagne or pie, with a side of sandwiches and a hot pudding afterwards, such as treacle tart or sticky toffee pudding.

Whenever the trolley came down the corridor from the kitchen to the dining room, the nurses would encourage the patients to line up for food. Clearly everyone was as excited as I was, because women would often push to the front and completely ignore the concept of manners and queuing etiquette. I grew so fond of the trolley man during my time there that sometimes he would let me stand behind the hot food with him and allow me to serve a spoonful of pie to the women. Thanks to being an annoying goody-two-shoes and sucking up to him, I was usually allowed extra custard once everyone else had been given their helpings.

If you picture being on a psych ward, you might imagine patients sitting in therapy circles or doing various activities. At first, I wasn't in a fit state to do any of these things, and nor were many of my fellow patients. Daily life on the ward mostly revolved around the staff keeping us out of harm's way, ensuring we took our medicines, and regularly assessing us for improvements. After breakfast, I would often ask to help the cleaners change out the bedrooms or follow the nurses around on their morning duties.

There were a couple of men working on the wards, although it was mostly women, and I gravitated towards their warm and calming energy. They never questioned my reality (which was, usually, very far away) and instead would ask questions about whatever I was telling them. This meant that I felt much safer and less fearful. When someone is manic, it can be unkind to keep hammering them with the truth. Instead, as I saw a lot with other patients in the extreme stages of psychosis when I was coming towards the end of my stay, much of your time in hospital is spent finding a nurse and explaining to them what you can see. A good, kind nurse is one who makes you feel safe. One nurse, who spent a lot of time with me at the start, would prompt me with questions when I was going off on one about God, asking me, 'Do your sisters like God too?' or 'Tell me about God!' In hindsight, I think this approach was so sweet.

Across my time in 'The Hope Ward', my delusions seemed to be based around a few key scenarios. In one, I believed I was on the set of *Casualty*. Perhaps this was my brain trying to rationalise why I would be in such a clinical setting. *You're not a patient – no, no – you're a TV director!* I would clap my hands and order my poor fellow patients to 'get out of my scene'. The other women, many of whom were experiencing delusions themselves, would sometimes obey my orders, or they would become quite frightened and the nurses would have to step in and pull me away or send me to my room.

During another delusion, which lasted several weeks, I believed I was flying to New York. Sometimes I would think I was in the departure lounge in the airport, while at other times I would demand that everyone pack their bags and I would go into other patients' rooms to check they were following my orders. In a similar vein, I wonder if this was my brain's attempt at escapism, to turn my depressing surroundings into something both exciting and familiar. My parents later told me how they watched me pack my bags in my room multiple times. Just like the nurses, they found it easier to play along with my reality than try to encourage sense and reason.

One particularly bizarre recurring delusion was that I had become the singer Susan Boyle. It's difficult to rationalise this one, because it did seem quite hilarious to everyone who visited me. I think, though, that my psychosis had brought up a lot of memories from my childhood, meaning my obsession with talent shows such as *The X Factor* and *Britain's Got Talent* bubbled to the surface. When I was young, I would print out pictures of all the contestants and stick them in a notebook, reviewing the performances each week. Before social media, I remember these TV shows being the hot topic I would obsess over with my friends, fuelling gossip for the week ahead. I think the re-entry of Susan, who had famously sung the *Les Misérables* hit, 'I Dreamed a Dream', on the third season of *Britain's Got*

Talent, represented the more childlike part of my brain making a reappearance. Susan was also notoriously misunderstood and judged before she started singing. Perhaps the manic me felt the same: people thought I was 'crazy' when I was, in fact, chosen by God.

Not mentioning the funny aspects of my behaviour in hospital would ignore a lot of my family's accounts of that time. Unfortunately, when you're that high, everything is hilarious, and you have complete confidence in whatever comes out of your mouth. My parents noticed quite quickly that my weird humour was soon to be a public demonstration.

When I arrived at the hospital, I was assigned to a doctor who introduced himself to me as Doctor TK. He would oversee my care, with weekly check-ins, and was responsible for deciding when I would be well enough to return home. Unfortunately, in this questionable headspace I latched onto his initials. Whenever he walked onto the ward, I would shout 'TK to the fucking max' before laughing my head off. No matter how many months went by, this joke remained absolutely hilarious to me, and there was nothing my parents could do or say without me repeating it over and over again.

I was one of the youngest women on the ward – the average age was probably around forty – and there was a diverse mix of ethnicities, life experiences and mental health problems. I was one of the more manic patients, unintentionally creating chaos in the communal areas on a regular basis. But there were also a lot of women who were down and depressed and mostly kept to themselves.

A few days after a woman from Hammersmith arrived as a new patient, there was much commotion around her bedroom as she had attempted suicide. From then on, a nurse always stood in her doorway. I later learnt that she had been in the system many times before – each time attempting suicide. This happened quite close to my discharge and frightened me a lot. I was still high at the end of my stay, but, as always, able to have mood swings. Earlier that day, this woman had been particularly funny in the communal area, speaking out loud to me and another young girl about her experiences. Aged only twenty-two, I had learnt very quickly that many people suffering from mental illness are unable to come back from it. I don't think I realised how much this affected me at the time.

The girl who was listening with me was only sixteen and was having anger issues after a break-up. Her violence had led to her having a daily check-in with the staff and only leaving each night after proving she was well-behaved that day. We sat opposite the woman from Hammersmith. She must have only been in her late thirties but looked exhausted and as though she hadn't showered recently or taken care of her appearance in a long while. She had cuts all up her arms, and I didn't know where to look or how to feel.

In some ways, the ward became more frightening towards the end of my time there. As I came back down to earth, I began to take in the traumatising effect that the other women's extreme behaviour was having on me. After the woman's suicide attempt, she occupied the room in seclusion that I had been in. I kept asking the nurses if she was OK, or if she would be in the end. I can't say that they could reassure me with much confidence.

She wasn't the only woman who had been in and out of the system. Some of the other patients had been receiving mental health support, in one way or another, for decades. Some had been there for solid chunks of months, even years. At the time, I understood that this was the norm for most patients. But now when I think about how many people stay in the system and never really leave it, I feel sad. When you're institutionalised, your illness becomes your life. Every day is about taking your medicines and speaking to nurses and doctors about how you're feeling. I can understand how that cycle can be difficult to escape from. Later on, this would become one of my biggest fears.

One woman in her sixties asked questions all day long. All we would hear throughout the day was: 'What time is breakfast?', 'What time are snacks?', 'What's my name?', 'Where's my husband?'.

I'm not sure what was going on in her world, but I do know that her husband would come to visit her every day and sit with her for half an hour or so, while she asked the same questions over and over again. She quite liked me, and one day she showed me her room. She had hoards of products piled high: loo roll, hand soaps, empty tissue boxes ... I think she was asking her husband to bring her the same things every day.

A few weeks before I was discharged, I was allowed to go out for half an hour every day with my family. I asked this woman if she wanted me to get her a chocolate bar. And so it began ... her daily Bounty.

The moment I got back, I would hear, 'Where's my Bounty?'

She would snatch it and walk off to her room, without so much as a thank you. Before long, more questions emerged. 'Will you get me a Bounty tomorrow?' 'Will you get me a Bounty today?'

Eventually the lead nurse on the ward told me I was no longer allowed to give her a Bounty, as it had become another compulsion in her day. I have awful memories of my last few weeks on the ward, remembering her face and screams when I told her I didn't get the Bounty. The nurses had to assist her into her bedroom, heartbroken and angry.

I befriended another woman who must have been in her mid-thirties. When we first met, she told me all about her children and her life with such clarity. Then a few days later she went into a full manic episode in which she walked around with her clothes tied into rags and attached to her pants or bra, her slippers hanging from her ears, or a T-shirt over her head, as if this was quite normal. She would dance towards the nurses with a completely straight face, making up chants and huffing and squatting. Then, she would play the drums on her stomach and sing loudly.

This kind of behaviour really didn't seem shocking on the ward. I was still, in my own way, trying to find meaning in everything. This woman took a huge liking to me and even called me 'the Messiah'! Sadly, our friendship came to an end when she started sharing my secret that I fancied one of the temporary night staff – one of the few men on the ward – who we will call K (but we'll come back to that later).

My best friend on the ward was a girl called Aaliyah. She was a similar age to me, lived in the bedroom opposite mine and felt like my ally on the ward. She was unbelievably funny, but also incredibly to the point. Her blunt comments (such as 'You're too ugly to model' and 'Your sisters don't love you') would sometimes make me cry.

We became friends at first because she let me message my friends from her Instagram account. My own phone had been lost somewhere in Stansted, which, in hindsight, was probably a good thing. I think I upset a few of my friends with messages in which I was essentially speaking in tongues, giving the impression that I was on another planet.

Aaliyah and I spent hours dancing to music videos on MTV in the living area, and I usually went to sit with her at mealtimes (although sometimes she would shout at me to go away). When I recovered enough to comprehend what was going on, I learnt that she had schizophrenia and was in and out of care after I left the hospital.

For a while, I tried to stay in touch with her, but our relationship became strained. Sometimes I avoided her – and at other times, she would send me abusive messages. Our friendship breakdown went beyond the usual issue of drifting apart or falling out and into the deeper emotions I have around my fear of relapse. I still feel very connected to her and our shared experience and incredibly guilty that I haven't been to see her. But I'm also too scared to reach out and repair things, because she is a reminder of what my life could be like, and my deep fear of regressing to how I was.

I have been living out in the world, campaigning to raise awareness and financially supporting myself. Her life runs parallel to mine but she's still unable to live a 'normal' life. It doesn't seem fair at all, and I'm not sure if I'll ever come to terms with that.

In the end, it took about four weeks for the anti-psychotic medicines to work their magic and pull me back into reality. I remember one turning point so clearly because it was the first time I recognised my mum when she came to visit.

I was messing around in the communal area, when one of the nurses said, 'Rosie, your mum is here to see you.'

As my mum appeared in the doorway, I thought to myself, *This is the most incredible sight I have ever seen.*

She looked adorable, holding an M&S bag full of blueberry muffins – my favourite since I was a child. When you're high, you can become highly conscious of people's energy and intentions. At that moment, I believed she was the kindest and most beautiful soul in the whole world. I realised just how much I had missed her. It felt like forever since I had seen her.

'Mummy!' I shouted as I ran over to her and gave her a hug. 'Oh my God, I love you so much.'

I cried, and she cried. It turns out that she had visited me every day since I came out of seclusion, but this was the first time I was present enough to acknowledge her existence. I can only imagine how relieved she felt too. She had watched her daughter orbiting another planet, wondering if I would ever come back down to earth.

When we went into my room, I suddenly felt so confused about where I was and why I was here.

'You have bipolar disorder, darling,' she told me. 'You've just been experiencing a manic high. Don't worry about anything though. It's all going be alright. You're safe, and we're all so proud of how well you're doing.'

When I first heard the word 'bipolar' uttered by that GP several months before, I was so depressed that a diagnosis sounded like a death sentence. However, being in hospital made it feel like a glimmer of hope. I was glad to have answers and reassurance that what I was experiencing wouldn't last forever and was being treated. Still, at this point, I wasn't well enough to take it all in.

I texted my best friend Maddie from my mum's phone with *BYE POLAR* and a laughing face. I thought this was really funny; it was such a silly word and its definition wouldn't sink in until later. On many occasions when my mum would visit, I would grab her phone. Whether it was to text a friend, or ask to see a picture of B, I would have moments when everything just made sense. Of course, my mum would make sure I didn't send any messages in that manic state. Especially when I often wanted to send B messages saying I loved him. My mum was protecting me, as she still does, from sending things to people in euphoria. Those messages are never a good idea.

My mum had been keeping in touch with my friends, updating them on my recovery, but thought it was best to keep my visitors strictly to family while I was deep in the throes of psychosis. I later learnt that my sisters had visited a few times, but they both found it very difficult seeing me there. I don't blame them, particularly as my parents have since shown me videos from week four, when I would stare into the camera and talk nonsense about monkeys. It's quite scary, to be honest. I find it hard to look at those videos, because I can't quite connect with that girl who looks dead behind the eyes. I find it tough to acknowledge that it was me.

Although I was starting to rediscover normality, it was still several weeks before I was deemed well enough to leave the hospital. In that time, I started to participate in some of the ward's activities, such as African drumming. My memories from this time are fairly vivid. I can remember ten people in a room banging drums with absolutely no rhythm – either completely manic, or worse, depressed. The woman who asked endless questions had the biggest drum, and she was banging it with no expression on her face. I think this was when I laughed for the first time – not from mania, but as myself. It was really quite funny.

Art class was another option that I took advantage of as I started to get better. We had integrated with the men's ward for this one and would all sit around big tables filled with pots of pens, paints and crayons. In many ways, it was just like being back at junior school. I created a painting for my mum, and a card for Maddie. I can't remember exactly what I made, but I'm pretty sure they were both made up of incoherent scribbles and probably went straight into the bin.

In my last few weeks on the ward, I was allowed to go out for lunch with my parents. I knew how to act like a 'normal' person and to ask the right questions: 'How are Amii and Lucy?' 'How's the cat?' 'How's work?'

I think these moments would give them hope that I was on the right track. But I was also still high, and the world around me would move in slow motion. I zoomed in on every footstep when the waiter brought over my pasta. The door to the restaurant would swing open with dramatic effect and then loudly click shut.

I told my parents about my visions. 'I've got magical powers. I'm not the same anymore.'

And they would know that I was very much not there yet.

Not long after, I saw Maddie for the first time. I was allowed to go out for lunch with her for a few hours. She had been so worried about me and was so relieved we could finally have a normal-ish conversation. I loved being with her, and it felt as if my old self was returning. I asked her about university and told her how much I loved her. We joked about the *BYE POLAR* message I had sent her at the start of my stay, as well as our conversations in the weeks leading up to me being sectioned.

When I had to return to the ward, it suddenly seemed so cold and scary in comparison to the outside world with my best friend. When I reached my room, I felt so upset that I couldn't spend the rest of the day with her. I realised how disconnected I had become from my friends. All my friends were still out there in the world – studying, dating, working, living. I was stuck here on this ward, and they would never be able to understand what I had been through. Not really. Reality crashed down on me. I couldn't believe I had spent the best part of two and a half months inside that tiny room, rather than in the real world.

I wasn't discharged from the ward because I was completely better. It was more because I could finally hold a conversation, I seemed 'stable' and was starting to be able to sleep, waking up at 6 a.m. instead of 3 a.m. at the height of my mania. My highs and delusions came in waves that were increasingly fewer with longer gaps between them. This was a sign that the worst of the psychosis was over and my medicines were working. And because I was ticking these boxes, I couldn't hang around – beds are limited on mental health wards. The hospital needed to hand mine over to the next person in need. It was decided that I was well enough for my parents to keep an eye on me from home, and I would be discharged to the intervention team near my parents' house for regular sessions.

Still, I viewed this as the end of my weird adventure in the mental health system. I was still riding high, but I knew who I was, where I was and what had happened (for the most part). I was ready to restart my life on the outside. When I was told I could leave, I was so excited – I couldn't stop thinking about my first Pret A Manger coffee and sleeping in my own bed. I told my mum and the doctors about all my plans to start modelling again.

When I spoke of my desires, I was met with sympathetic looks and told not to expect too much, too soon. I was too high to handle their negativity. I waved goodbye to my fellow patients and the nurses, and I skipped out of the heavy-duty doors with my parents, armed with prescriptions for lithium (for my mood) and aripiprazole (for the psychosis).

I might have bipolar disorder, but it's all under control now! I am cured! I am healed!

Reader, I was not.

5
hello darkness, my old friend

My first week at home was like a dream. My bed, in my parents' house in London, had never felt so warm and comforting, especially in comparison to the hard, plasticky mattress in the hospital. My appetite was completely bottomless, so I devoured my mum's home cooking, going back for second helpings of roast chicken, mushroom risotto and fajitas. Hospital was behind me, and my future stretched ahead, glittering with exciting opportunities.

Yes, I was still as high as a kite.

But even in the sickly-sweet glow of post-hospital life, I felt very conscious about how much I had missed. I had been gone for three months, in which time a new coffee shop had opened up around the corner. I had no idea what had been happening in the news, what new music had been released, or whether my friends in relationships were still together or had broken up. Maddie had started a master's degree exactly when I was sectioned, and I arrived home to a letter from her, telling me how her first term had gone.

It was disorienting to have missed such key events in my friends' lives. It felt as if I had just woken up from a very, very long sleep. As a result, I was keen to make up for lost time and immediately messaged all my friends (from a brand new phone) and made lots of plans to catch up.

One of my first arrangements was with a friend I knew from modelling. She came over to our house for a home-cooked roast, courtesy of my parents. I was so excited to see her and discuss all my plans to get back to work.

When she arrived, she gave me a hug and handed me a candle and a card. 'I hope you get better soon,' she had written in the card. It was a kind gesture but my heart sank. As we ate our food, I tried my best to act as normal and happy as I could, but I felt a sudden crash. I kept thinking: *What do you mean, '...get better soon?' I am better already!*

Clearly no one believed this – except for me.

In that first week, I was in complete denial about the state of my mental health. It began to hit home when my mum drove me to my first meeting with my intervention team, one week after I left hospital. Ideally, I would have gone sooner – but the hospital respected the fact that I needed a break from medical professionals before diving head-first into my treatment plan.

I thought the treatment for my bipolar was done and dusted. In reality, it had only just begun. My hospital stay was all about pulling me down from a manic high. The mania itself wasn't my mental illness – it was only the most extreme symptom. My doctors had told me while I was still in hospital that during the next stage of my treatment I would need to learn to manage the rollercoaster of bipolar in the real world – essentially to avoid another manic episode and hospital stay. My dad had been doing his research and told me that 25 per cent of bipolar patients never need to be sectioned again. The goal, everyone said, was to be one of them. At that point, I was still too high to understand what this all meant.

My first meeting took place in Westbourne Park, in a sterile, clinical room that instantly gave me flashbacks of my time on the ward. It was a frosty November morning and the room wasn't well-heated, so I could feel my toes turning icy inside my trainers. Mum and I sat opposite a team of six people, who each explained their role in my recovery. They would be here for me every step of the way, they said, for the next three years.

Three years?! I thought. *Why would they assume my recovery will take that long?*

I now understand that this is a rough period of time that the NHS uses to help integrate mental health patients back into normal life. It means that, during this period, you have constant access to support, rather than being discharged straight to the GP system (like the general population). This is an amazing part of the healthcare system, designed to ensure that the most high-risk people receive the help they need. I am fortunate to have been in London, because the quality and accessibility of care varies depending on where you live. At the time, though, it felt as if I had only just escaped prison, so this is not what I wanted to hear.

My team was made up of two psychiatrists, a therapist, a care co-ordinator, a nurse and a trainee psychiatrist taking notes as part of her university course (which made me feel as if I was being studied – not the best for morale, I can tell you that much). The care co-ordinator explained that she would be my point of contact, available whenever I needed her over text message. She was a small Scottish woman, who wore glasses and radiated nervous energy.

I later found out that this was her first job as a co-ordinator, and it would end up being her last. I would come to be very fond of her, but I'm not surprised the job wasn't for her. She had a very anxious disposition and always looked as if she was going to cry. Given her role involved being on the receiving end of heavy information, I can imagine it took its toll.

The psychiatrists and nurse were there for any medical check-ups I would need, including regularly testing my blood to ensure I wasn't receiving poisonous doses of lithium. One of the psychiatrists was a jolly woman who must have been in her mid-50s. When I was high, I could be sensitive to people's energies – and her cheerful energy made me warm to her instantly. She began the meeting by calmly reminding me about my bipolar diagnosis.

Although I had been told about it a few times while I was in hospital, I still wasn't sure exactly what it meant. I had been diagnosed with bipolar 1, which is defined by manic episodes that can last for several days and are so severe that a person needs urgent medical care. Apparently, doctors knew unequivocally that they were dealing with bipolar 1 when I first arrived in hospital. I was told my manic high was a 'textbook' sign, thanks to the spiritual delusions, intense energy and hallucinations that came in waves. The psychiatrist told me that the depressive episodes that usually follow these manic highs can also last for lengthy periods of time.

As a result, their main focus was on monitoring my medicines. At this point, they wanted to wait for the lithium in my system to start working.

'I can assure you that this is the best medication for patients with bipolar 1, for reducing the risk of suicide,' the psychiatrist said.

Hearing that phrase, I became frightened. *Why would I be suicidal?!* I didn't want to hear this. I wanted the team to tell me that I would recover quickly, I wouldn't need any more meetings, and to send me on my way. Instead, they told me that recovery would be 'a marathon, not a sprint', with a lot of trial and error. They said that I would need to have two meetings a week for the next few months with different members of my team – and if I needed to speak to my care co-ordinator in person or on the phone, I could have a further two days.

This was extremely worrying. I couldn't understand why they were being so negative about my recovery. It felt as if they were expecting everything to go wrong. I began to tune out what they were saying and let my mum take over with any questions. She could sense I felt overwhelmed, so she reached over and held my hand. It was all too much. As soon as we got in the car to drive home, I burst into tears.

After we had walked through the front door, Mum asked if I wanted to talk about it, but I shook my head. I threw myself onto the sofa, switched on the blow-heater – aiming it directly at my feet – and turned my attention towards *Married at First Sight UK*. I didn't want to think about my diagnosis or depression or suicide or therapy. I wanted to watch strangers get married to each other, and all the drama that came with it.

Over the next few weeks, the reality of my situation became sharper. I had made lots of plans with friends, but I felt anxious when people asked the natural question, 'So, what's next?' Whenever they asked me that question, I would panic and feel unable to respond.

I wanted to go back to modelling, but my agent had told me to take my time getting better. 'We can touch base in the new year,' she said. I was sure that the weight I had piled on during my hospital stay had something to do with it.

At first, I enjoyed seeing my friends. But those interactions were fragile, because we weren't hanging out in the way we used to. It was different because I was the centre of attention. Everyone was so glad I was back. Initially, I regaled them with my ridiculous tales from the ward, such as the time another patient did a poo in my sink. But eventually the novelty wore off (for both me and them).

I realised how disconnected my life was from theirs. They were still working hard and partying all night, just as I had been before my episode. But me? I was spending my days going back and forth to medical appointments with my mum. She had hardly worked since I'd been in hospital, and I felt guilty that her diary revolved around my care.

I wanted to give her a break and be around my friends, but the gulf between our lives made it hard. I felt as if they would never understand what I had been through. My negative thoughts slowly ate away at my post-hospital positivity, until there was very little left. Still, I had one glimmer of hope: Christmas was coming up. I was looking forward to my friends taking time off from work and studying, and I hoped the festive joy of the season might drag some of that positivity back.

Sadly, the opposite was true. Christmas is a funny old season. It can be the most joyful, treasured time. But when you're struggling – whether that's with grief, mental illness or anything else – it can serve as a reminder of all the joy you're lacking, and everything you've lost. Over Christmas, I sunk into a deep depression. I was constantly tired, lacking the energy to even play a game of Monopoly, let alone do any form of exercise. My appetite was bigger than ever, and I remember sitting on the sofa on the evening of Christmas

Day, conscious of my rumbling stomach, wondering why I still felt hungry after having eaten almost non-stop during the late evening. Everyone around me was saying how full they were, and I couldn't understand why I was so disconnected from both my mind and my body.

My family and friends, sensing I was miserable, kept telling me: 'Next year is a fresh start. 2019 will be your year.'

But then I would go to my doctors' appointments, and they would say, 'The real work starts next year, as this is when we'll get you managing your bipolar.'

I kept thinking: *I don't want to start next year. It sounds like hell.*

Suffice to say, I started January without much excitement for the year ahead. I felt like crap. And it was at this time that I started experiencing issues with my therapist. The majority of my meetings were with the psychiatrists and nurses, focusing on my medication. But I was also assigned a therapist, who I was supposed to see for the next two and a half years. Let's call her Miss R.

My relationship with Miss R must be one of thousands of cases of a patient being paired up with the wrong therapist. I'm willing to accept some accountability on my side, though. I didn't exactly go into our sessions with the best mindset. Our meetings were scheduled fortnightly, giving me the impression from the outset that this was the least important part of my care. Added to that, I already felt let down by therapy. The woman I had been seeing privately throughout my depression in 2018 was lovely but hadn't caught my bipolar when I was on the cusp of a manic episode. And then there was the fact I was fully depressed by the time I started my sessions with Miss R. I had little trust or faith that a therapist could help me. When I was high in hospital, I would natter non-stop to the nurses about my life. By comparison, in early 2019, I didn't feel like speaking at all.

At our first appointment, while I was sitting beside my parents, Miss R seemed fairly cold but polite enough. She was extremely slim and wore several layers of clothing to keep warm. She had printed off worksheets, and I was told to jot down what my 'triggers' were. At this time, the word 'trigger' was quite alien to me, so I had no idea what I was supposed to say.

The most memorable worksheet – which I would end up filling in for several months – was my mood chart. I had to describe my mood out of 10 every day (1 being the most depressed; 10 being the happiest), dividing the day into five separate sections – for example 'waking up until 10 a.m.; 10 a.m. to lunchtime; lunchtime until 3 p.m.'

During those first few weeks, the number only peaked at 3 on the days when I didn't have to speak to any mental health professionals. 1 1 2 2 1 tended to be the most prominent pattern; it would go up to 2 around lunchtime when I would sit on the living room floor catching up on *Married at First Sight UK*, smoking my vape and drinking hot Robinsons squash. My vape had become a new habit during my depressed days – it gave me a small, two-second hit of nicotine that sadly became the highlight of my day for some time.

I hated all the exercises Miss R made me do – I dragged my feet and groaned every time she initiated a new activity or worksheet for me to complete. But in the new year, I thought I would try to get something out of therapy. I was feeling extremely hopeless about the state of my career. I had signed back up to work at the start of January. But turning up to a modelling shoot looking lifeless, I received feedback that I was 'no longer selling clothes like I used to'.

Savage. I was also much heavier than I used to be, and I spiralled into self-hate, believing that my weight-gain meant the end of my career and my world. The combination of not working, living with my parents and seeing mental health professionals three times a week made me fear for my future.

How long would I feel like this – perhaps forever?

I thought I could solve this by getting back to work. And to do this, I needed to get my body back to how it was. I was adamant the medicines were the culprit for my increased appetite and inability to exercise. I believed that these were preventing me from getting back to my normal life.

Arriving in Miss R's office on a cold January morning, I decided to open up about my concerns. I told her that I was struggling with bottomless hunger, and I believed this was making me more depressed because it was ruining my chances of returning to my career. I told her how I had become obsessed with curry – gorging on delicious cheese naan and curry sandwiches – and the crash that would come the next day, when I would feel guilty for eating so much in one sitting.

I wanted reassurance and understanding – even just an ear to listen to my concerns would have been great. Instead, what I got was, 'If you want to speak about your eating disorder, you'll have to find another therapist. We are here for your bipolar.'

I was shocked and upset. I immediately felt ashamed. It was as though my concern was inappropriate and I shouldn't have raised it. And so began several weeks of therapy that made me feel even worse. Over our next few sessions, she would tell me that modelling wasn't a real job, that it had likely caused my illness, and that caring about my weight was self-indulgent and pointless, seeing as modelling was a career I shouldn't return to. Her tone was patronising and scary, and I retreated into myself more and more in every session we had together. I often left the room crying. Whenever I felt hungry, her voice would pop into my head, telling me I was silly and privileged for even thinking about such things. She kept mentioning how 'lucky' I was in our sessions, making me feel as though my current predicament was simply a result of my character: that I was ungrateful and vain.

I knew she had some fair points about my job. Having such an image-focused career probably wasn't ideal for my bipolar recovery. But insisting that my depression was something I had brought on myself through the work I had chosen, rather than helping me find tools to manage it, felt like a personal attack – especially to my fragile mind. Eventually, I broke down to my parents and told them that my sessions with Miss R felt as if I was being bullied. With their support, I terminated my relationship with her. Later, I filed a formal complaint about the way she had treated me. Sadly, nothing ever came of it – as is often the case, unfortunately.

Of course I know that therapists are only human. They won't always get it right, and you won't always click with the person you're assigned to. But the whole situation was extremely upsetting. Having since read a lot about bipolar and its ability to be comorbid with other illnesses, I now know that it's normal for binge eating (or anorexia) to go hand in hand with bipolar, especially when you throw the impact of certain medicines into the mix. Miss R was right in saying I had a problem, but her dismissal of its importance, and how badly it was impacting me, left lasting scars. It reinforced the idea that I shouldn't open up – not even to someone whose job it is to listen without judgement. The process scarred me so much that I stayed away from therapy altogether for another five years.

Sadly, this is the case for so many of us. We have one bad experience with the wrong healthcare professional and it can prevent us from seeking the help we need. It was a useful lesson, though. I would now encourage anyone who finds themselves in a similar position to trust their gut when it comes to their treatment. Regardless of Miss R's judgement of my career and my personality, I would say that going straight into talking therapy after hospital wasn't the right approach for me. It was too much, too soon, and I struggled to open up for a long time. All I cared about after hospital was returning to 'normal', and therapy made me feel anything but. Waiting outside her room for my appointments, my whole body would seize up. It's a shame that therapy didn't work out, because I know how life-changing it has been for many people with bipolar. But I also know that finding the right therapist can take time. If your therapeutic relationship isn't working, it's OK to say so.

With therapy out of the equation by spring 2019, I was in a depression so deep that I wondered if I would ever escape it. The main focus of my treatment centred around medicines and getting the balance of chemicals just right. It didn't feel like my meds were working; if anything, the side effects appeared to make me feel worse. I have already mentioned the extreme hunger and binge eating, which became a defining feature of my life. My skin worsened due to all the junk food I was eating, causing me to further spiral into self-hate and low self-esteem.

Then there was the relentless exhaustion. Depression causes fatigue all by itself, but the medicines that are used to soften highs can make things worse if the dose isn't right. During this time, I woke up in the morning at around 10 a.m., feeling too tired to even shower or brush my teeth. I was so spaced-out even when I was awake, and found myself wishing the time away until I could sleep again. Sometimes, I would try to nap in the afternoons, but actual sleep never materialised. Instead, I would lie down and stare into thin air.

These side effects – alongside heart palpitations, trembling, migraines and brain fog – led my doctors to make tweaks to my medicine combinations. It went something like this: *Let's reduce a dose here. Let's increase the dose there. Let's try this new medication – but it will take a few weeks to work, so we'll need to wait before we see improvements.*

Every time they suggested a new three to four-week wait time, I felt as if I was being pushed to my limit. Did they not understand the urgency? The whole process was exhausting, and I know my parents were just as frustrated as I was that nothing seemed to help.

I became reliant on my parents once again, just as I was as a child. Mum would brush my hair in the mornings, because I had no energy to do it myself, and then she would tuck me into bed at night, as the thought of another day made me feel shaken and scared. My parents would try to take me out for coffee – something I had always loved – but I would just sit in silence, unsure of what to say. Often, I would cry while I ate dinner with them because I couldn't believe how something so simple could highlight how low I felt.

My poor parents bore the brunt of my sadness. I once again became Clingy-Childhood-Rosie; I only really felt comfortable around my mum, but I also felt guilty about how much of her life had become revolved around me. This was the second time she had had to give up her life for an ill child, and it hurts to think about the toll that must have taken on her. Still, she was infectiously positive and always tried to find small ways to cheer me up, even if that was just playing with my hair while we watched TV on the sofa, or taking me to the supermarket where she would let me load up the trolley with my favourite yoghurts.

In early 2019, my parents went on a skiing trip with some friends of theirs, and my sister, Amii, came to the house in West London to stay with me. I wanted them to be able to have a break, but I couldn't help calling my mum several times a day. When they returned, I felt unbelievably relieved. I realised that 'separation anxiety' isn't just something people say; it was a real physical and mental issue I was grappling with. The girl who begged her parents to allow her to board at school, and lived abroad when she was only 18, seemed far away. I felt that I had regressed to the most dependent version of myself. I wondered whether I would ever be independent from my parents again.

I should also say that I know I am incredibly fortunate to have such unflinching parental support. Family support is considered to be a key marker in a person's recovery from psychosis, while a lack of a solid support system is known to increase the likelihood of relapsing to a manic episode. Miss R would remind me of this often; she was right, but her tone wasn't so kind. In my state of mind, I could barely recognise my own face, let alone my immense privilege. Looking back, I am extremely grateful I had them to lean on.

Mum had pretty much stopped working to be with me, but as the accountant for my parents' business, and the composer for any music within the adverts they produced, she still had to work for a couple of hours every day at her desk. During this time, I would lie face-down on the sofa in their office near our house, while I waited for them to finish working. On one particularly sad day, my dad walked into the room to see me in my usual routine: head in the crack of the sofa, inhaling the crumbs and dust. Quite a sorry sight, really.

'Rosie, mate, why don't you go and get some fresh air?' he suggested. 'Maybe you can take some pictures while we're working, and then you can show us your photos afterwards?'

Before I became ill, I was passionate about film photography. I took my camera everywhere; I loved catching my friends smiling candidly or capturing the scenery of beautiful places. Sometimes, I would walk for hours around London just to clutch my camera and finish a roll of film.

In that moment with my dad, I had never felt so lonely and so far from myself. I wasn't that Rosie anymore – that wide-eyed girl who could see the beauty in the world and wanted to document it. I was the opposite: the world was devoid of beauty. It had all sunk into the black hole of my mind. I knew that my dad had suggested this activity in the desperate hope that it might spark something, that maybe I would remember who I used to be. But it just didn't seem possible to me – that Rosie was gone.

'No, thank you,' I said, choking back tears. 'I'll just stay here.'

He sighed and left the room.

I realised my dad was grieving the daughter he knew, before depression stole her away. It broke my heart.

* * *

Sometimes, my mind was completely empty. The thoughts I did have tended to be repetitive and negative, like a TikTok video that just keeps playing when you leave your phone open. Most of these thoughts could fit into two broad categories: fear and self-loathing.

My biggest fear was the unknown. I didn't know anyone personally who had been diagnosed with bipolar 1, so I was forced to look for guidance on the internet. I wanted someone to tell me that I would never end up in hospital again, that this dark cloud I was living under would pass, and that there was light at the end of the tunnel. Instead of quelling my fears, good old Google made them infinitely worse. I scrolled through thousands of forums and comments from people with my diagnosis, talking about the hellish side effects of medicines – and documenting their first, second, third or even fourth manic episodes. Even worse, I felt haunted by all the talk of repeated suicide attempts. *Was this my inevitable future?* Absorbing this information – which seemed easier to read than a book, or even a magazine – made me feel more hopeless than ever.

I was terrified that I had lost the old me altogether. That girl who loved snapping pictures of her friends ... was she dead and gone? My depression convinced me that she was. Nothing interested me anymore. I remember looking at my mum's bookshelves and thinking: *Why does anyone bother reading? It's all pointless.*

I used to love shopping, planning my outfits and getting dressed. At the height of my sadness, I would wear the same thing every day – a pair of boyfriend-cut jeans, a tank top and a thin navy cashmere hoodie that my mum had recently bought for my twenty-third birthday. This forced my mum to check if I had showered. Eventually, she would start leaving clean clothes at the end of my bed to get me to change. Sometimes, when the pressure of my fatigue prevented me from even sleeping, I would watch videos of my old self. I hoped I would find some answers; some key back to who I was. Instead, I found myself unable to relate to any of that girl's mannerisms and acts of confidence. It was like watching someone else entirely.

Modelling seemed like a distant daydream. Not only was my self-esteem at rock-bottom thanks to my appearance, I also knew that I had lost a key part of what had made me a successful model: I had been bubbly and chatty. I know that a core reason why brands would book me again and again was because I could fill the room with energy and make everyone have a great day on set. Now, I was the opposite; I could suck the energy out of a room like a Hoover. My self-worth had been tied to my career for so many years, and now it felt as if I would never be able to go there again.

When I told my mum about this, she said: 'That's okay, we can find something else you're passionate about ... when you're ready.'

But my world had revolved around mood charts, medical professionals and pills for so long. Would I ever be able to work and support myself? How would I ever find the courage, determination and motivation to try something new?

I was also scared that my sisters and friends had lost patience and understanding with me. I worried they really thought, deep down, that I was only acting this way because I wanted attention. Even today, this inner voice loves to creep in whether I'm tearful or struggling to cope. This is one reason why I tend to keep my darkest thoughts to myself. Sometimes, my illness makes my thoughts so extreme, they're almost unbelievable. *Why would anyone believe me?* These moments feel especially lonely. It's awful to feel misunderstood or disbelieved. This wasn't anybody else's fault – it was my mind tricking me into thinking I was completely alone.

Then there was the self-loathing, which felt engulfing. Slowly I was processing the label that would be attached to me forever: 'bipolar'. In my mind, this was a word I associated with being crazy or broken. And to be honest, I *felt* crazy and broken. So it was difficult to believe 'bipolar' could be anything but a death sentence. The depression made me harsh on myself. *You're always so miserable – everyone hates you,* the little voice said. *You look disgusting. No one will ever hire you, and no one will ever love you.* I was angry with bipolar for robbing me of my job, my personality and my life.

This made me incredibly jealous of those around me. I had never considered myself to be a jealous person before, but depression made me green with envy. I hated anyone who was able to live their lives without this kind of disruption. Social media reaffirmed the narrative I had created that everyone else's lives were perfect.

They don't know how lucky they have it, I thought, *to be free and doing whatever they want, earning money, going on holidays, being relaxed.*

I was even jealous of my parents in their sixties, because they were able to go to bed and escape me and the storm cloud I carried on my back. Me, on the other hand: I was stuck in the endless grey.

On the rare occasions I accepted invitations to see my friends, I would be able to act happy for five minutes at the start, then quickly feel overwhelmed and burst into tears and need to leave. When I could speak, I was unable to talk about anything other than my illness, which was often met with silence, as most of my friends didn't know the right thing to say or do, or how to act.

I think the reason I would always have to leave was that every time I saw my friends, I was reminded again of how different our lives had become. If I kept quiet and listened to them speaking, the smallest thing would set me off. If they complained that they were tired, the anger inside me would rise up. *YOU THINK YOU'RE TIRED?!* I would want to snap, weighed down by the heavy doses of medicines. Or, if someone complained about work, I would want to scream: *AT LEAST YOU DON'T HAVE TO LIVE WITH YOUR PARENTS AND YOU CAN WORK!* Of course I kept these thoughts to myself, but it was a horrible feeling having that negativity seep into situations I used to love being in.

It was a vicious cycle. I hated talking about other people's lives – which were all so much better than mine – but I also hated being the centre of attention and the subject of everyone's concern. It felt as if I was being watched, judged and studied all the time – by medical professionals, by everyone – and yet I was completely incapable of thinking about anything outside of my sad and sorry life. Eventually, every kind of conversation frustrated me. I didn't know what I wanted. I didn't want to be alone, but I didn't want to be around other people either. I just knew that life felt noisy – both inside my head, and outside of it. All I wanted was silence.

By May, suicidal thoughts had made their way into my repetitive thought rotation – and they got louder every day. I had lost hope of ever getting better, and I felt so guilty about what I was putting my family and friends through. I began to stash medicines in my room, rather than taking them. I was beginning to feel comforted by the idea that my life would be over soon. I started lying to my mum because I didn't want her catching on to how I was feeling. I cried silently at night, hoping she wouldn't hear, and I watched her smile as I ranked my mood above 3 on my chart (when, in reality, I was feeling -10).

On one lovely sunny day, I went to Boots to pick up a prescription for anti-nausea medicine (a fun new side effect from an antidepressant my doctors were testing out).

'This is a two-week supply,' the pharmacist told me. 'You'll need to speak to your doctor if the sickness hasn't subsided by then to get a new prescription.'

I nodded, while the voice in my head murmured, *It doesn't matter, I won't still be here in two weeks.* The confidence of that voice shocked me and scared me.

The next day, the weather had warmed up. Mum insisted that I come with her to visit Lucy at work in the city. We bought salads and sat cross-legged in the park. The boiling weather made me sink lower than ever; the fact that even sunshine couldn't elevate my mood made me feel inhuman and hopeless. I was wearing the same outfit that had become my uniform for the past three weeks.

While we ate lunch, I had the impression that Lucy was feeling frustrated by the extended timeline of my recovery and the lack of improvement in my mood. I was paranoid that she hated me, for taking up so much of our parents' time, for being a drain, for ruining everything. I really believed, in that moment, that I was the biggest burden on my family. I thought that everyone would be so much happier if I wasn't there.

Mum noticed I hadn't said a word over lunch, so she suggested we go shopping to buy some new jeans on the way home. All I wanted was to be alone again and crawl into bed, so I simply responded with a pained look (yes, even shopping had now become terrifying for me). I looked at Lucy and couldn't quite read her expression. Was it confusion? Anger, even? I assumed the worst and burst into hysterical tears. My life had become so unbearable, and I was dragging everyone in it down with me. Mum agreed to take me straight home on the Tube. Lucy tried to hug me, but I was in too much agony to respond and tensed up in response. Mum held my hand as I hyperventilated while we rattled through each station.

The voice in my head telling me to take my own life had become loud and unignorable. As soon as Mum opened the front door, I darted for the stairs and fell on my way up. I screamed – a huge, guttural scream. I couldn't keep it in anymore.

'I don't want to be alive,' I confessed to her through choked tears, after she had led my shaking body to the sitting room. Weeks of suicide ideation had bubbled to the surface, and I really felt that it was my last option.

She cradled herself and cried on the sofa, while I sat on the carpet, unable to look her in the eyes.

The sun was brighter than ever, streaming through the shutters of the sitting room. Life should have been good – everything was right in the world, except for me. After talking to me for an hour, terrified by the depths of my despair, Mum called my intervention team for an emergency meeting.

This was rock-bottom.

6
the bumpy road to recovery

The next day, we sat opposite my care team in that same clinical appointment room where we had first met seven months before. Both my parents came along this time, and I noticed a momentous shift in their demeanours. My mum and dad had been positive and cheerful throughout every stage of my recovery so far, but this was the first time I saw them angry – really angry.

I shrank into my chair – shaking, tearful and embarrassed – as my parents shouted at the doctors, furious that we hadn't seen any improvement despite constant medication adjustments.

'Why is nothing working?' my mum demanded. 'We need a sense of urgency here; we're running out of time.'

In that moment, I felt more hopeless than ever. *My parents' lives would be so much easier if they didn't have to deal with me*, the little voice said. *I'm ruining everyone's lives.*

My team seemed just as dumbfounded that everything had gone so wrong so many months after my discharge, so they decided to refer me to a specialist psychiatrist at a different hospital for a second opinion. While I waited for my appointment, they said I would be placed on 'suicide watch', which involved having two visits a day from the emergency intervention team – one at 10 a.m., and one at 3 p.m. – to check in on me. Since I had confessed to Mum that I'd been stockpiling my meds, it was decided that they would also bring me my medicines, to ensure there were only ever small quantities in the house. A few days later, I went into my parents' bathroom to look for a spare loo roll to find that medicines of any kind had been cleared away and hidden. I felt heartbroken by just how serious things had become.

It was strange to suddenly be under constant surveillance. Of course, it had been this way when I was sectioned, but I was too high to notice how intrusive it was. When the nurses visited me twice a day, the speed at which they spoke reminded me of how people talk to cats. It was laughably depressing. I thought, *Wow, I can't believe my life has reduced so much that I am now, in fact, a cat.* I knew I had brought it on myself, but this only made me feel increasingly worthless. Clearly, I was incapable of living as a normal human being.

For as long as I can remember, my powerhouse mum has spent her days writing music for the company and organising the finances. But fearing for my life, she stopped working altogether, and my dad worked from home more often to ensure there was always someone watching me. I can barely tell you what happened in this time, but I just remember trudging through the days, feeling inexplicably heavy. I hardly said a word while I watched reality TV, my mum squished next to me on the sofa gripping my hand as if I might evaporate.

I noticed that her temperament had changed. Rather than being optimistic about the doctors' trials, she understood that she would need to take matters into her own hands, and she became determined to get me better. In an attempt to shake things up a bit, she took me to sit on our flat roof one afternoon. It was possibly not the wisest choice for someone who is suicidal, but she had a plan. She told me to shout and swear as loud as I could for a few minutes.

It was an interesting approach, since I had been essentially mute for several days. But I followed her instructions, and it felt like the whole world came bursting out of my throat as I screamed into the sky. A few birds flew out of the trees, clearly terrified – and a baby started crying somewhere in the distance. It was so ridiculous that I actually started to laugh. My mum looked at me, and we both sat there laughing on the roof.

After we came down, my mum made me a cup of tea and explained that the nurses were considering sectioning me again. While the first time hadn't been a choice, this would be. We discussed the decision that evening and decided to hold off. The thought of not being around my mum again felt too risky, as she was the only person who could make me smile. I was worried that being readmitted to a ward would push me over the edge.

Thankfully, a major glimmer of hope was on the horizon. When June rolled around, I could finally attend my appointment with the new psychiatrist. She was based in a different hospital to where I had been sectioned before; this time, we were in Central London (rather than in the suburbs). On entering a hospital again, seven months later, it felt as if my health was being taken seriously once more, and I could sense that my mum recognised the importance of that too.

After a few minutes in a large, clean waiting room, we were called in to speak to the psychiatrist. Before we even had a chance to explain the suicidal ideation I'd been having, she began to apologise.

She flicked through my notes, saw the months and months of medical trials, and expressed her concern that I hadn't been treated properly.

'You should have been seeing improvement by now,' she said.

I could see the palpable look of relief on my mum's face. She hadn't been 'crazy' for shouting about my care – she was right. I felt relieved too. I knew that none of it had been working. I just didn't know how to fix it.

Very quickly, the psychiatrist told us about a new 'miracle drug' that had been helping people to manage the most extreme forms of bipolar.

'Quetiapine – it's an anti-psychotic with mood-stabilising effects,' she explained.

I had tried countless different medicines, but the word 'miracle' felt profound – and not just because I have a propensity towards grand, spiritual, God-like thoughts. Finally, a medical professional seemed confident in a specific treatment. So far, my care had been all about throwing shit at the wall to see what stuck. Returning home armed with a new prescription, I dared myself to dream that things would be different this time.

My parents seemed to feel as hopeful as I did. Instead of hanging around waiting for the medicine to kick in for the billionth time, they suggested we escape London for a while and stay at the house in Gloucestershire. My care team agreed that I could stay in touch over the phone from there, hopeful that I could have a break from the repetitive depressed cycle I had found myself in (at the very least).

The first few days in the countryside were more of the same – heaviness, reality TV, a hit of nicotine from my vape, lots of food, sleep, Robinsons squash. And then, about two weeks after starting quetiapine, that promised miracle arrived.

At 9 a.m. on one bright Saturday morning, Dad suggested that I come with him to grab a newspaper from the local supermarket. As we walked, I noticed a café on the left that I hadn't seen before. I looked through the window and could see people eating huge plates of eggs, sausages and baked beans.

Without thinking, I asked, 'I've never noticed that café before. Have you ever been there?'

As pathetic as it sounds, this simple comment represented a breakthrough. I had just asked my dad a question without thinking what to ask. The words had simply come out of my mouth. I was genuinely interested in his answer (he had been), and I felt engaged in our conversation ('What did you eat?'). I noticed that I didn't feel trapped in my own mind, alone with my depressive thoughts.

Once we had picked up the newspaper, I was so excited to tell my mum what had happened.

'Mum, I asked a question and had a conversation, and it didn't make me want to die!' I announced as I burst through the front door. It's probably not the kind of thing a parent expects to hear from their twenty-three-year-old daughter, but I know she understood how much of a milestone this was.

That day, the future didn't feel so scary. In fact, I wanted to talk about it. At dinner that night, I spoke about my next steps after getting better (I wanted a job, which we all agreed shouldn't be modelling). For the first time in a long time, I could imagine staying on this planet, and maybe it wouldn't be so awful. I wrote a '6' in my mood chart for the first time. It felt as if I had been underwater for a long time and I was finally coming up for air. I could feel the depressive voice in my head becoming quieter – and a more positive one was making a comeback.

Over the coming weeks, my mood lifted gradually each day. It was a feeling I hadn't experienced in more than a year: content and calm. For so long, I had yo-yo'd between depression and grandiose, over-excited thoughts. It was unusual to find myself somewhere in the middle, but my God, I wasn't complaining.

One day, I woke up and decided to go for a run. I put on my headphones and clicked 'play' on the 'Run Faster, Bitch' playlist my friend had made for me years before. It was a lovely selection of club music and feel-good noughties bangers. (I still believe 'Knock You Down' by Keri Hilson is the world's best track to run to.)

My whole body ached while I ran. It had been so long, but the music filled my ears and I felt fully present. I didn't think about the purpose of the run, or how unfit I was. I just hummed along and focused on my feet hitting the floor in that familiar (albeit slower) rhythm. When I arrived home, I hopped in the shower and remembered how good it felt to wash after exercising, soaking away the sweat and inhaling the grapefruit-scented steam.

If you've ever experienced depression, you'll understand how groundbreaking these tiny moments felt. When you're depressed, everything is covered in dark smog. Nothing feels nice, nothing feels enjoyable, and everything feels pointless. If you have ever emerged from that thick fog, you'll know that it can feel as if you're experiencing the world for the first time. Honestly, it's beautiful.

Much to my mum's delight, I started caring about personal hygiene again. I stopped lying that I had brushed my hair and teeth (I actually did it because I wanted to) and I even started moisturising my face. My routine of sleep-eat-TV-repeat had become unsatisfying, so I started accompanying Mum to the supermarket to buy ingredients for dinner. I started thinking about recipes I could make for her and Dad, and for the next few weeks I became resident chef in the house. I had a new ritual: preparing dinner and blasting music in the kitchen. I could actually spend some time alone without being afraid of my own mind.

It wasn't all rainbows and butterflies. I would still wake up low in the mornings, feeling heavy and lacking in purpose. But I started being able to help myself, prioritising movement, and enjoying the taste of coffee again. By the afternoon each day, I felt more positive. Within six weeks, I had stopped thinking about ending my life.

Without a doubt, my life had improved massively. But I couldn't say I was 'better' just yet. I was adamant that my full recovery was dependent on my independence. My parents had been incredible, and I leaned on them so heavily, but I knew I could only be a 'normal' twenty-three year old if I moved out and got a job. If I could just get a nine-to-five, I wouldn't have to spend so much time in my own head, bored and navigating recovery care.

While we were still in Gloucestershire, I filled my days between running and cooking with scanning job websites. I wasn't particularly fussy – any job would do – but I came across a posting for a field sales manager at a brand-new kombucha company and decided to apply. Kombucha – a kind of fermented juice – is everywhere now, but it felt quite trendy and modern in 2019. I didn't know exactly what the role would entail, yet I decided it would be perfect for me.

Health is important to me! I'm good with people (or at least I was)! I'm going to live the super cool start-up life – just like any other independent twenty-something!

I met with the founders the following week in London and somehow managed to charm them with my limited knowledge of kombucha and passion for sales (fake it until you make it, right?). A couple of days later, they told me I got the job. I was so excited and ran downstairs to tell my parents about this milestone news. They were happy for me, but my mum wanted to ensure I kept my feet on the ground.

'That's great, Rosie,' she assured me. 'But remember you're still recovering. Try not to pin all your hopes on this role, OK?' (How did she know me so well?)

***

While I waited to start my new job, the stars aligned that my friend, Moya, was looking for a housemate to move into her flat in East London. We had met while working for the same modelling agency, but she was also studying at university in London. I hoped that moving in with a friend would give me the push I needed to start becoming my old self again.

I was buzzing to make this step but also terrified. My life had revolved around my care and my parents for almost a whole year by that point. I didn't know if I could handle being away from the two people who knew me best, and who had no choice but to love me unconditionally. Of course, Moya knew about my bipolar – and she had been so supportive – but no one except my parents knew the extent of it. I felt vulnerable knowing that a friend might have to witness Nightmarishly Depressed Rosie in action.

Mum dropped me off at my new flat the day before I started the new job. I felt like a kid again being dropped off at boarding school (except far less confident than I was in those days). Moya helped us unpack my boxes, and we chatted about all the fun things we would do while we were living together. It made me feel much more at ease, but I still panicked when my mum left.

'You can always come home, Rosie,' she said, noticing the panic in my eyes when I saw her out the front door. 'You can call me any time. We're always here.'

That first night, Moya had a date round at the house. I awkwardly third-wheeled, sipping my soup dinner, while they drank prosecco and laughed on the sofa. They offered for me to join them, but I felt embarrassed and weird, so went off to my room to get my stuff ready for my first day at work. I also called my mum, even though it had only been about two hours since she had left. This would become my pattern for the next few weeks – calling her once every few hours. The separation anxiety was real. I still had phone calls with my team every day, but I had managed to reduce my in-person meetings (they supported the fact I had started working).

My expectations of working at the kombucha company went something like this: exciting, fast-paced, with super-cool colleagues in a snazzy office. But the reality didn't quite match up. First of all, I hadn't considered that 'field' sales meant being out and about ('in the field', so to speak), which meant my role consisted of carrying heavy boxes of kombucha around London in granny trolleys to pubs and restaurants. It was quite the baptism of fire. I had barely spoken to my friends for months, and here I was, having to speak to complete strangers.

My job was to get the owners to try the drink (not too difficult), before encouraging them to order some (quite a bit harder). In my first fortnight, every single restaurant I visited accepted the samples, but not one wanted to place an order. Given the role was very numbers based (and there was commission to be earned), this wasn't ideal. I was absolutely exhausted at the end of each day, lugging around my bottle-filled trolley without anything to show for it.

Perhaps unsurprisingly, I slipped slowly but surely back into a depressed headspace. *Is this my life now?* I thought to myself every time I showed up to the trendy East London office to collect more stock. *Am I totally useless at everything? What's the point in me?*

Moya came home from uni every day to find me watching *Married at First Sight* (the Australian version, this time) on the sofa. She would come and join me, grabbing a surplus bottle of kombucha from the fridge. She was always kind, but I couldn't help feeling like a burden. And so, while she went out partying every few days, I mostly escaped back to my parents' house to be looked after. I felt safer there. I didn't have to pretend that I was 'better' and everything was fine.

It was during this time of flux – living in a new place, working in a new job – that I started dating my former nurse. For that to make sense, we need to rewind for a moment.

Do you remember I said that I fancied one of the temporary night workers while I was in hospital? Well, 'I fancied him' was a bit of an understatement. I truly believed I had fallen in love with him. Let's call him K. Most of the nurses were female, but he was one of the few men who worked on the ward. I say this because I think it was rather like when you're in school, and everyone has a crush on that one younger teacher. As you get older, you realise they weren't really that amazing – they were just better than everyone else and in a position of authority. Add some grand spiritual delusions into the equation, and you have the perfect storm for a somewhat tragic love story.

When I picture my first interactions with K, the visuals aren't exactly realistic. He shone like a star against the dismal surroundings of the ward. He was about twenty years older than me, but he was sweet and, in my manic state, I believed he was the most beautiful man I had ever seen. My grandiose thoughts had led me to believe that Bill was the love of my life on the day I was sectioned. After a few weeks, that same belief in fate and soulmates had transferred over to K.

Later, he would tell me about his first shift with me. It was two weeks into my stay – the height of my mania – and I was refusing to keep my clothes on. Apparently, I was sitting on the windowsill – unable to sleep – and I kept pulling my trousers down, smacking my bum and laughing hysterically (absolutely mortifying). He had been instructed to sit in a chair in the doorway of my room, as I was threatening to jump out of the window or run away. This part, I do remember. I thought he was my guardian angel.

After a few weeks, my medication started working. I told him about my break-up, my family, my hopes and dreams. He was inquisitive and pure and asked me questions as if I was completely sane, even though I often spoke in riddles loaded with religious imagery. His presence became the highlight of my stay in hospital. I looked forward to his shifts more than anything, and I truly believed that our meeting was destined.

MAYBE THIS IS WHY I'M IN HOSPITAL! I thought. *TO MEET THE LOVE OF MY LIFE!*

At one point during my stay, I didn't see him for a few weeks – and I became terrified that he had only been a voice in my head. But then he returned (it turned out he'd just gone on holiday).

'I'm in love with K,' I announced to my mum on one of her visits towards the end of my stay.

She batted me away, hopeful that this obsession would dissipate along with my mania. Of course, it's extremely unethical for a nurse to pursue a patient (especially a much younger one); there's a power dynamic and duty of care that would make any kind of romantic relationship wholly inappropriate. And I have to clarify that K kept this boundary with me. That is, until a few months after I left the ward, when I managed to track down his personal contact details.

I was deeply depressed, but the memory of our conversations and his light that shone brightly in my darkest hour kept me going. I thought that maybe if we were reunited, I would feel better again. I pondered whether my depression would become more manageable if I was dating someone really kind and caring.

I made it my mission to find him online, and I reached out on social media.

At first, he was very resistant to talking to me. 'It's not appropriate, Rosie,' he said. 'I was your nurse.'

'But you don't even work in that hospital anymore – and I'm better now!' I urged him, weeks later, once the quetiapine had begun to work its magic.

Eventually I wore him down, and he agreed to meet up for coffee. When I saw him again, I was immediately reminded of those hopeful, meaningful nights on the ward, where he would stay up with me for hours. I felt instantly comfortable around him. It felt as if he understood me, even in my most chaotic highs and torturous lows.

I thought I could hide my instability from K as we went on several dates, from smoking shisha in North London to a late-night curry in Hampstead Heath. Talking and finding out more about him, the rose-tinted glasses gradually faded. When I told my mum I was dating him, she was furious.

'Rosie, it's completely inappropriate. I can't believe he's pursuing you,' she said. 'You're an adult and you can do what you want, but I really don't think this is right. I am not speaking to you about this – you know the right thing to do.'

I didn't want to disappoint her, especially as she had given up her whole life to care for me. With her voice ringing in my head, I started to view things differently. Add to that, I was sinking deeper into a depressive episode – hating work and unsure about the future of my life – and realised that this new relationship wasn't helping anything. It just made me feel more confused. He was so much older than me, and our lives were worlds apart.

When he came to our flat and Moya cooked us a stir-fry, I knew it was never going to work. He sat on the end of my bed as I cried and told him the twenty years between us was too big an age gap, and the timing wasn't great given my depression was coming back. I remember this moment quite clearly, as the bed broke when he sat on it – surely planks breaking beneath the mattress was some sort of sign that it wasn't meant to be.

'I understand, Rosie,' he said as he got up and left the flat. 'Look after yourself, won't you?'

Looking back on that experience now, I can't help feeling embarrassed and ashamed. It frustrates me to think that I can't always tell the difference between reality and delusion. I was so sure, even as I was getting better, that this man was my destiny – and I even managed to convince him that I was right. When you have bipolar, it can be hard to tell the difference between genuine love and hypomanic obsession – but we'll come back to that in Chapter 10.

Only three weeks after moving in with Moya, I decided to temporarily move back to my parents' place. I had ended my fated romance with my former nurse, I was unhappy in my job, and depressive thoughts were creeping back into my everyday rotation.

> *I thought life was meant to get better – so why is it becoming even more complicated? Has the quetiapine stopped working? Is there any hope for me?*

When I attended a regular meeting with my intervention team, I told them how I was feeling (I neglected to mention the relationship with K, though).

'Give it time,' they reminded me. 'Recovery doesn't happen in one linear line. You have already come so far, but it's normal to feel like you're going back a few steps every so often.'

In the meantime, I still had to work. That week, I had to help out at a stall for my company at a food and drink fair in London, encouraging people to try samples and buy bottles. During a cigarette break with my colleague (aka my nemesis – who was the same age as me but making sales left, right and centre), I confessed that I might have to quit my job soon, because my mental health had taken a turn. The next day, I discovered that she had bounced straight to my boss and relayed the news that I hated life, my job and kombucha.

The founders called me into their office, and I was swiftly fired. At least the decision was made for me.

But then came the dreaded question: *What the hell am I going to do now?*

7
rediscovering rosie

So there I was, back home again and depressed about the direction of my life. But this time, with the 'miracle drug' coursing through my body, I felt determined that I could find a way through this low period. I just had to find my calling. I decided that all I needed was a purpose to help me get up each day.

Dating K did have one silver lining: it reminded me how much I appreciated and respected my nurses while I was in hospital. While living on the ward, I had idolised the nurses who had shown me so much kindness and security when everything else was topsy-turvy. They were such selfless beings, who had given so much of their time and energy to support my recovery.

I thought: *If I could focus my energy on other people, perhaps I wouldn't be so consumed by my own illness.* I can't remember the exact moment I had this epiphany. I think it was when I was scrolling through never-ending job postings, thinking, *None of this feels right*. It came to me in a split-second and I decided to act on it impulsively. *I'm going to become a nurse!*

Before I even had time to speak to my parents about it, I had submitted applications for several university courses to study mental health nursing. I knew it was a snap decision, but I felt so sure that it was the right one. (Again, very difficult for me to tell the difference between a bipolar impulse and a genuine brain wave.)

Not long after, I was called in for an interview to study at a top London university. The interview experience was terrifying, and I sat on my hands while I attempted to push through the discomfort of the questions they were asking me.

'Why are you applying for this course?' one of the interviewers asked.

I quickly realised that I didn't have many reasons, except for the fact that I had experienced a psychotic episode myself, and I was in awe of the work that mental health nurses do. (I kept the details of my episode vague, and skated over how recent it was.)

'I think I'm in the perfect position to help patients, because I know what it's like to be hospitalised,' I said, channelling as much confidence as I could.

'How will you cope with the stress of university and managing your bipolar?' another asked.

I explained that focusing on a goal helps to keep my most severe bipolar symptoms at bay. If I'm honest, I had no idea if this was true – but I hoped it would be.

Somehow, I managed to convince my interviewers that I would be perfect for the course. A few days later, I found out I had secured a place for that September (just a couple of months later). I felt so excited that my life was about to take a new direction – a direction that made me feel good about myself, as if I could make a difference. My intervention team weren't particularly enthralled by the thought of this, and my parents seemed a little nervous too. One nurse suggested that perhaps starting the following year would be more realistic, given that my first attempt at resuming a nine to five job had just failed. I was so offended and determined to prove her wrong.

I didn't know it at the time, but I would never become a nurse. In fact, I wouldn't even attend one day of lectures. Regardless, the seed had been planted and I had given myself something to work towards. Knowing that I had something secured for September, I gave myself a permission slip to enjoy my summer without incessantly worrying about my future. Feeling much better, I moved back in with Moya – who was on her university summer holidays. And it was during these summer months that I made huge strides in my recovery.

There was a heatwave that July. London's parks were full of sunbathers and little children eating ice lollies. Besides some pre-course prep, there was nothing else I needed to do – so it was the perfect time to find my way back to myself. With the sun shining down, like a good omen, I became obsessed with music again. Even though my choices were slightly depressing – my playlist was full of Liz Lawrence, Sufjan Stevens and Sylvan Esso – it reignited a passion that reminded me of my old self. When it was very hot, Moya, her friend Nima and I would get on the train to Hackney Marshes with towels and lie in the sun listening to music all day. Head leaning on my hands, sun on my back, I noticed that I didn't feel lonely anymore.

My friends became extremely important to me during this time. Over the past year, I had lost some friends. There's nothing like a mental health crisis to weed out the people who aren't meant to be in your life. But it also made me more grateful than ever for the people who stuck around. I was in awe of Moya at that time, and we became inseparable. She had been so consistently kind to me, and I appreciated it more than anything. She backed up any view I had, complimented me all the time, and picked up little sweet treats for me on the days I struggled. With a uni crowd around her, Moya would often have friends over in the evening before going out clubbing – and the hushed voices would always go silent around 10 p.m. when she knew I took my medication to sleep. Little by little, she helped me believe I wasn't a burden.

I began to accept more of my own social invitations, too. Seeing old friends didn't feel quite as taxing as it had before; I wasn't jealous of their jobs and lives, because I was starting my own path soon. I found myself increasingly able to talk about topics outside my bipolar – I became interested in the world again. I tentatively started drinking alcohol again, too. That said, I had been told this could interact with my medication, so I kept drinking to a minimum.

I found it easier to be around my closest friends than with wider groups of people I didn't really know. My mind often darted around, making it hard to stay present, saying things such as: *What do they think of me? Did they only invite me out of pity? Do they think I'm boring because I'm not drinking and leaving early?* Sometimes I'd get home to Moya or my parents and burst into tears, terrified that whoever I went out with hated me. But the more I did it, the easier it became.

My close friends understood, and no one put pressure on me to drink or stay out late. I was normally in bed by 10 p.m. after every social event, as opposed to my usual pre-illness time of 5 a.m. Still, it was progress. Each night I arrived back home from a social gathering, exhausted and slightly overwhelmed, I felt proud of myself for going in the first place.

Among the glimpses of a normal girl in her twenties, I started dating again. One week, I had an epiphany that I should DM anyone from my sixth form I had ever found attractive. I decided this would be a great way to ease myself into dating – reaching out to people I already knew seemed less daunting. I received a reply from one fit guy I had been in geography class with, and we organised a date on a Thursday night. Within minutes, I realised we had zero chemistry and the attraction vanished – but I pushed on anyway. After a few more drinks than I should have had, I stumbled home to Moya and a bowl of cereal.

We laughed about the awkwardness of my evening while I danced around the room to Jack Johnson. I curled up in bed that night beaming, despite the fate of my date, blissfully unaware of the wave of depression that would accompany my hangover the next morning. *I was alive and young! Dating was normal! And I was doing it!* It's hard to describe how special this felt.

There were still mood swings; days where I felt so overwhelmed that I would travel back to my parents' house in floods of tears. But the good days outweighed the bad, and I had started to acknowledge the transience of my worst emotions. I had learnt by then that my bipolar was a bit like jumping on a trampoline – I might go down, but I'll ping up again. Eventually, I could spend more than a week away from my parents, and I relied less on my mum's phone calls. I slept better in my new bed. I was grateful for every moment of this. That's one positive of hitting rock bottom: you can recognise the good when it comes and remind yourself to live in the present.

Another breakthrough in my recovery came when I rediscovered reading. I hadn't read a book since my trip to India with B, until one of my school friends gave me a copy of *This is Going to Hurt* by Adam Kay.

'It's so easy to read – you'll love it,' she told me – and she was right.

Lying on our balcony, I raced through the book, laughing and relating to so many observations of life in hospital. And so, a new hobby was born. I became obsessed with uncovering books that would help me learn more about mental health. Many of the books I read were terrifyingly negative (we'll go into more of that later), but even the most depressing accounts made me realise that everyone's experience with psychosis and bipolar 1 is so different. I became curious to learn more about my illness on my own terms, rather than trying to run away from it and pretend it didn't exist. Even now, I still turn to reading, especially when I am in a low, to pass the time and take me out of my mind.

Soon enough, September rolled around and it was time to start my university course. I had been added to a WhatsApp group of my fellow students and had an induction day, and then I was invited to come and collect my 'outfit' for the year ahead. So far, so good. But while I was still on campus, I tried on the nurse's outfit and looked at myself in a tall, slim mirror in the changing room. I immediately realised that Nurse Rosie wasn't meant to be.

The uniform took me back to my time on the ward – a time that I hadn't yet processed or made sense of. The nurses had been the best part of my time there, but I was still absolutely petrified of my bipolar, and the idea of being anywhere near a hospital inpatient ward made me feel sick to my stomach. Looking after people in the grips of psychosis, doing night shifts, and working for hours on end without rest ... it would be a recipe for disaster. I could finally see that, clear as day.

I called my mum's number. 'I'm dropping out of uni,' I said when she picked up the phone.

Funnily enough, she had been expecting this call, although I don't think she expected it quite so soon.

Ignoring the messages in my university group chat discussing freshers' week events, I hopped on a bus back to my flat, knowing full well I would never set foot in that university again.

I didn't feel sad about this realisation. If anything, I felt more motivated and galvanised. Nursing wasn't the right path – that much was abundantly clear – but turning my mental health crisis into something positive still mattered to me. I couldn't deny that my interest in mental health was growing stronger and stronger. I was probably on my eighth book on the topic. I just didn't know how to convert my passion into action.

Knowing I wouldn't be able to afford to rent my room unless I had some income, Moya suggested I come with her to a meeting at my old modelling agency (where she was still working). I knew that modelling wasn't the long-term goal, even though it had once been my whole identity. My agency said they would love to have me back, so Moya and I celebrated with Aperol Spritzes. I felt as if my friend had sorted me out for now. We didn't know what the future had in store, but at least we had each other.

A few weeks later, I had another epiphany while I was in the shower washing my hair. *Viva Fever*, my brain announced, as if by magic. As soon as I dried off, I set up an Instagram page with the same name. I didn't actually know what the page would be. A walking club? Somewhere to organise a run with friends? Whatever its fate, I decided

I would use this platform to raise money for mental health charities. I might not be able to physically support people as a nurse, but I could use the skills I did have to make a difference.

I messaged my sister's friend, an illustrator, and asked whether she could help me make a poster for my first event. And then, a few days later, I shared it with the caption, *Let's walk from Angel to Victoria Park next weekend – please donate £5 to Mind to join.*

An hour before the proposed start time for the walk, I sat nervously outside a restaurant in Angel, eating breakfast with Moya.

'Even if it's only us, chick, it'll be so nice,' she encouraged me.

We paid the bill, and she told me how proud she was of what I was doing as we walked towards the meeting point.

As we turned the corner, I felt my heart stop in my chest when I noticed two school friends chatting away in their leggings and trainers. As I walked towards them, they ran up to me and gave me a massive hug. I burst into tears, so taken aback that they had shown up.

Next, a girl I didn't know tapped me on the back. 'I'm here for the Viva Fever walk,' she said. Her name was Katherine. I couldn't believe someone I didn't even know would want to come along.

Ten minutes later – with a group of fifteen girls, made up mostly of people I knew – we set off down the canal. I spoke to Katherine the whole time, as I felt so grateful she had come along without knowing anyone. I was still too scared to tell her what my diagnosis was, or my story, but I asked what had led her to join me that day. She told me how she had been sectioned for dissociation – and she was only one year older than me. I couldn't believe it.

Maybe what I went through was sort of ... normal?

The next day, I went to work on a shoot. As I had my make-up done, I couldn't stop talking to the make-up artist about the walk. I still felt buzzing from the day before and couldn't wait to explore what else I could do with Viva Fever.

A few weeks later, I decided to put on my first speaking event, to raise money for the mental health charity Mind. I reached out to two speakers who could share their stories of mental health, and I also enlisted the help of a school friend to create a poster for me. When I posted it online, I was terrified that I wouldn't manage to sell out all forty seats in the East London venue I had found. I did sell out in the end and, if I'm honest, it was mostly from people I knew personally. But it was a great start, because the cost of the tickets all went directly to Mind, which made me feel that I was doing *something*. I had never organised a charity event before, so it felt a little bit like fumbling around in the dark. My mum – saint as she is – spent two days helping me make canapes.

When the day arrived, and the room started filling up, my anxiety turned to excitement. Having sipped on a few drinks before people took their seats, I was a little tipsy and hyper when it came to introducing the speakers. Having now interviewed a lot of people over the years, I've noticed that I tend to embarrass myself or say something very personal to the other person, so they feel they can relax and do the same. This was probably quite a heightened version of that, as I launched into a monologue about why I had started Viva Fever. I blurted out that I was grateful for everyone who had remained friends with me after I believed I was Jesus, before proclaiming that the event had 'Jeremy Kyle vibes' thanks to the way I had staged it to interview the speakers one by one.

Nonetheless, the speakers were so professional and engaging, and the evening was such a success. Everyone stayed afterwards for a while, chatting and discussing the stories they'd heard. Afterwards, my friends joined me for a night out nearby and I kissed a boy I'd been on a date with who had come to the event. It definitely wasn't your usual charity event – getting a bit too drunk and snogging someone – but I still felt proud of what I had produced, and I couldn't wait to plan my next one. This energy translated well to my modelling work, too. I received great feedback and started feeling good about myself.

By the end of 2019, life wasn't perfect, but I was edging closer to some form of normality. I was earning money and planning more events to help raise money for different mental health charities. But you'll know by now that what goes up must come down. As I entered 2020 feeling more hopeful than I had in years, I didn't know that a whole world of sadness was waiting for me. And this time, it wasn't all in my own head.

8
the light behind trauma

From the outside, my life was beginning to look similar to how it was before the Great Downward Spiral of 2018. I was working regularly on modelling campaigns and socialising with friends. But I definitely wasn't the same person as I was back then.

For starters, I was much more sensitive and insecure. A work trip to Gran Canaria for a shoot caused a doom-spiral because I believed the photographer hated me. I was back in a consistent running routine, but my appetite still hadn't slowed down, and I would find myself secretly bingeing and then feeling huge amounts of shame. I confided in Moya about what I was experiencing, but I still managed to hide the worst of my overeating episodes from her. When she went out for the evening, I would run to Tesco to buy four packets of Creme Eggs and several boxes of granola. This would trigger a crashing low mood the next day, during which I felt exhausted and disappointed in myself.

There was clearly a problem here, but I didn't want to raise this with my doctors when I had just begun to reduce my interactions with them. I told myself that this hangover from my illness would go away if I could just have some self-control. So, the days after an evening of overeating became increasingly extreme – I'd push myself to run long distances, or have twenty-four hours of only drinking coffee. On these days, under-fuelled and over-exercised, I felt high. I appeared giggly and energetic, proving that bipolar highs don't necessarily signal happiness.

My sleep worsened, thanks to worrying about putting on weight and hating my job. I was running off a fragile kind of energy, desperately trying to be OK and prove to everyone that I was better. Despite my outward projection of happiness, I was beginning to confront the fact that bipolar was a lifelong diagnosis, and I'd have to deal with my turbulent mind for my entire life. I felt that I was hanging on to normality by a thread.

I'm not sure when exactly the words 'Covid-19' and 'global pandemic' entered my vocabulary, but it felt like they appeared from nowhere – and then suddenly they were everywhere. I know that this was an incredibly scary, stressful, traumatic time for many people. But for me, personally, the announcement of a nationwide lockdown in March was a godsend. My agency told all their models (who were mostly teenagers) to go back home to their parents' houses to wait out 'the next few weeks' (of course, no one really knew at that point how long it would last).

Speaking to my fellow models, many of them felt panicked about being out of work. But me? All I felt was relief. I knew I was still so unwell, and masking it had become unsustainable. I knew that I needed to be back in Gloucestershire with my family; all I wanted to do was curl up on the sofa and be around people who knew me (and my bipolar) inside out. My sisters came home too, wanting to escape London and feel supported by our parents. It was the perfect excuse to turn inward again and focus on my recovery.

I was very flat in the early stages of lockdown, particularly because my overeating got out of control. With almost nothing else to do, I ate. Easter weekend was particularly hard. As embarrassing as this is, I felt my stomach grumbling in bed at night, so I went downstairs and ate everybody's Easter eggs in one sitting. Filled with shame, I slept in until the next afternoon – while my family wondered where the hell all the chocolate had gone. When my mum confronted me about it, I cried and shook and admitted to someone else properly for the first time that the hunger due to my medication was causing me so much unhappiness.

It didn't help that I drank more, too. Like many families in lockdown, evening wine (or cocktails) became part of our routine, and I didn't want to miss out. Feeling tipsy while sitting on the sofa was nice, but then the next day I'd wake up with a sinking feeling in my chest. After a day of feeling sorry for myself, I'd go back on my over-exercising, clean-eating mission – and then the cycle would repeat itself.

I don't think this experience was unique to bipolar. The lack of a normal routine seemed to mess everyone up a bit. All my friends seemed to be drinking and eating more, and everyone had taken up running since all gyms had closed. It sounds bad, but I actually enjoyed the fact we were all in it together. I chatted to my close friends on Zoom every few days; there was a communal spirit that made me feel less alone than in my previous lockdowns-for-one. I was no longer the focus of every conversation. We all had our own struggles with being at home, from the lack of work to the annoyance of being with family. We were all bored and frustrated by the uncertainty.

There were silver linings, though. My eldest sister, Amii, gave birth to her baby Dennis just a few months before lockdown. Our family unit strengthened as we all huddled around this new arrival. Lucy was the only one who could work normally, so she had shut herself away in the attic at her desk before joining me for an early evening walk around the village.

I have to be honest, Covid-19 itself wasn't something that scared me. My biggest fear was losing my mind, and this fear extended to the people I loved. Those closest to me hadn't been able to spot my dangerous descent into psychosis, so I found the invisibility of mental ill-health petrifying. I was aware that my happiest friend could be in the thick of a breakdown and I wouldn't necessarily know. In my mind, Covid-19 felt like a much more obvious threat. There were things we could do to avoid it. There were constant conversations about it. There was no stigma attached to the type of person who caught it. Of course, the threat was very much real, but my fears simply didn't lie here.

Unfortunately, just a few short weeks later, my biggest fear became a reality, when I lost one of the most important people in my life.

Siôn had come into my family's lives ten years earlier, when he struck up a relationship with my sister, Lucy, during her uni years. Like most relationships around this age, they were casual for a while before Lucy felt ready to introduce him to the family as her official boyfriend. I remember all of us nudging her about this new mystery man she was always texting and calling when she came home for the holidays, until she felt ready to introduce him.

Eventually, Siôn came to stay in Gloucestershire for a long weekend. Wrapping Lucy up in his arms on the sofa, he had this incredibly relaxed energy and charisma – and we all loved him instantly. He became known in our family for his sense of humour, his ability to speak fluent Welsh (which he would occasionally burst into, without any of us understanding a word) and his unendingly optimistic outlook on life.

I never knew the ins and outs of their relationship, but it was obvious that he adored being with my sister, and she adored being with him. Over the course of their time together, I noticed a change in Lucy; she became more relaxed and spontaneous than she had ever been. After university, both of them began working in the high-pressure finance world, so they moved in together in London.

As young children, Lucy and I were inseparable, despite the non-stop arguments. I have memories of us playing in the garden together, making dens, or huddled up next to each other at a computer playing *Sims* or *Rollercoaster Tycoon*. On family holidays, we took our Nintendo Game Boys to a corner away from my parents and would roll on the floor laughing for hours on end at our inside jokes. Every weekend or holiday was made special by having my sister at my side.

During our teenage years, we drifted apart. It wasn't something I had worried about, but having Siôn around helped to bridge the gap between us during the years around my diagnosis. I sometimes squeezed onto the sofa to watch *Made in Chelsea* with them, or was third-wheel for dinner at their home. He showed me that the three of us actually had a lot in common, despite our very different career paths at this age.

Soon enough, he became a constant at every family event. Throughout all my most chaotic, depressed and anxious episodes, Siôn felt like a rock to me. It was borderline impossible to feel miserable around him, and he would make small gestures that made me feel less alone. He'd send messages such as *So good to see you, Rozza!* after every family event, or he would call me randomly on a Sunday morning. Later, Lucy would tell me just how much my psychotic episode had affected Siôn, how tearful he was when it happened, and the fact he constantly asked about my progress. For Christmas in 2019, he bought me a book of jokes for people with mental illness. At the time, I just thought he was being his upbeat, thoughtful self – always looking out for me, and helping me to see the funny side. But the next year would bring to light his own struggles.

Before the pandemic hit in 2020, Siôn had temporarily moved to San Francisco for an exciting work opportunity. I didn't know much about why he was there, or how long for, but Lucy would frequently update us that he was missing his family and us, despite loving the outdoorsy aspect of his new life. Lucy had always been fiercely independent, and she seemed confident that their long-standing love could stay strong despite the distance.

One day in early May, Lucy came downstairs from the attic where she had been working, looking as pale as a ghost.

'I'm worried about Siôn,' she said as she burst into tears. She had just been on the phone to his new flatmate, who told Lucy that Siôn had slipped into a worrying depression. He was concerned about Siôn's swift decline.

Hearing this, my heart sank. Siôn was pure sunshine. I couldn't comprehend him being in such a dark place. I tried not to get too involved in the conversation, because I was afraid my fear would be palpable. I knew that I could be triggered by any mention of mental ill-health, and I didn't want to freak Lucy out, or make it all about me.

After talking things through with my parents, Lucy decided that it would help Siôn to have a few weeks off work; coming back to London and staying in their flat, just the two of them, would do him some good. Within days, he had been signed off for six weeks, the flights were booked, and my parents drove Lucy back to London (despite lockdown rules) to greet Siôn back at their flat.

I was desperate for updates about how Siôn was doing, but I didn't want to overwhelm Lucy – and I know she only really wanted to speak to my parents while she focused on supporting Siôn. Still, I sent her texts every few days:

> *I really think you both should come to Gloucestershire so we can all be together. Please send my love to Siôn!! No need to respond. I miss you both xxx.*
>
> *Thinking of you. Please tell Siôn that it gets better, even if that feels impossible. He is not his thoughts xxx.*

Rather than receiving direct responses, I overheard pieces of information in dribs and drabs from my parents. Taking leave from work made Siôn feel hugely embarrassed, and he began to feel paranoid on top of the low energy and flatness. He was worried that people were after him and that his life was about to fall apart. This made me particularly scared, because I knew how powerful these delusions could be.

I'm not entirely sure how quickly things escalated, but I know that Siôn's mum moved into their flat for a few weeks to ensure he was in good company while Lucy worked. A GP had prescribed antidepressants, but nobody felt Siôn was showing extreme enough signs to be sectioned.

He'd had a year of bad mental health when he'd started uni, but in recent years he had been known to all his friends as a beacon of light. I think everyone hoped it was a blip – a result of homesickness and the chaos of change during a pandemic. I noticed that Lucy would become angry over the phone whenever anyone tried to offer advice. Now, I understand that she was deeply afraid that Siôn wouldn't survive the extent of his illness.

By the end of May, it seemed that he had turned a corner – at least, he stopped voicing his most distressing thoughts. He was reading books on mindfulness and smiling in any photos Lucy took of him. His mum moved back to Wales but still insisted on calling every day. I have since understood that he wasn't really better at all; he was simply convincing everyone that he was fine to be left alone. On 1 June, while my sister had popped out to the shops for just a few minutes, Siôn died by suicide in their bedroom.

My dad was the one to call me and tell me what had happened. He and my mum had seen Lucy and Siôn the day before for a picnic, and they were in the car driving from London to Gloucestershire when Lucy called them. Clearly, he was so shocked that he was unable to deliver the news in the 'right' way. I picked up the landline in the kitchen to hear the words that would return in my nightmares: 'Siôn has killed himself.'

I can safely say this was the hardest moment of my life. I thought the universe had already dealt me and my family a few difficult cards, but everything paled in comparison to this. Looking out into the sunny garden, I rushed out onto the grass and fell to my knees. I didn't recognise the sound that came out of my mouth. It was a piercing scream that travelled through my entire body. I felt physically in pain as I rocked myself back and forth.

Amii's husband, James, was home when it happened and ran outside to see what was going on. He fell to the ground to join me as I told him the terrible news. We clung onto each other as time seemingly stopped. My understanding of the world shifted to total confusion. *Siôn was always so happy and well. How could everything have gone so terribly wrong?*

Over the next few weeks, our primary goal as a family was to take care of Lucy. She moved home in a thick fog of pain and trauma, and we took every day as it came: making sure she was eating, finding trashy reality TV to watch, and giving her space to scream and cry. We received a flurry of beautiful texts, cards and packages from people who had come into contact with Siôn. It was testament to his infectious energy that he'd had an impact on everyone he met.

It's strange to admit it, but the intensity of emotion from losing Siôn sent me into a high. In the same way my break-up triggered my manic episode, I have learnt that I don't always have 'normal' reactions to extreme emotions. My brain works differently, and the only way I can rationalise it is that my brain attempts to protect me from trauma. It's a coping mechanism. Plus, I hadn't been sleeping – feeling sick with worry for Lucy – and I now know that lack of sleep is a trigger for hypomania. I became impulsive and decided that a date was in order – immediately.

At this point in 2020, lockdown rules were easing. Many of my single friends were starting to date again with the new-found freedom, and I somehow thought it would be a good idea for me to do the same. I went to stay with Moya occasionally (who had just moved back to London) to give Lucy quality time with my parents, and on these days I scheduled back-to-back dates on Hinge.

I went to meet one particular guy at his flat in North London. As soon as I met him, I knew he wasn't my type, but my hormones were flying all over the place. Sipping on a martini at 3 p.m., I listened to this man boast about his rooftop yoga sessions and his 'eclectic' music taste. He was distinctly uncool, but every time he offered me a crisp, I could feel my lust growing stronger. It was extremely confusing, experiencing such an ick for someone but my body telling me otherwise. This was my first experience with hypersexuality – which I had read can be caused by hypomania (we'll come back to this).

'I need to leave, otherwise I'll have sex with you,' were my exact words as I stormed out of his flat. I'm sure it's a date he'll never forget, poor man.

Going high as a result of pain continues to confuse me just as much as it did then. More recently, one of my closest couple friends suffered a miscarriage while I was with them. I managed to stay calm and drive them to the hospital, but the following day I pinged up into such a high that my boyfriend at the time hadn't seen before. Running 10 km and then finding him *so* attractive I couldn't keep my hands off him – it's a reaction I'm still embarrassed about and don't want to identify with. I know that my reactions aren't always aligned with how I'm feeling, and I recognise how difficult this is for loved ones to contend with. It's not 'normal' to be buzzing with energy after something awful has happened. It's not 'normal' to act happy when you're horrifyingly sad. It's not something I want, but I'm increasingly recognising this incongruity as part of my life.

I still feel hugely guilty for speaking to Lucy about my dating life (an ill-advised attempt to distract her). It upsets me when I think about how inappropriate that was, when she had just lost the love of her life. I wish I had kept my mouth shut. But I also learnt a lot from these moments. I'm now better at recognising my own reactions, and I try to spend time by myself when I'm high. I'll go on long runs to shake off the energy and write down my bizarre hypomanic thoughts, rather than inflicting them on other people.

Despite the high, there were some triggering moments over the next few weeks that brought the pain into sharper focus. On one particularly difficult day, a delivery van pulled up at the house in Gloucestershire, while only Amii and I were home. It was Siôn's suitcase from San Francisco that had been sent back to the UK. It didn't feel right for us to receive it; I couldn't bear to think what Lucy would do with it. Amii and I cried for hours while watching trashy TV. We could barely say anything to each other. There was simply a shared understanding of how awful it was: that Siôn's suitcase sat in our hallway, and he wasn't here anymore to unzip it.

Siôn's funeral was also a horrible day. It took place in Wales and, with restricted capacity thanks to Covid-19, only my parents could accompany Lucy. His favourite T-shirt had been a tie-dye pattern, so almost 200 people gathered outside the church wearing a similar one. I wore mine in London, sitting in tears in my friend Ella's garden while flicking through pictures of the funeral online. It was unbearably painful, but also felt like a beautiful way to honour his vibrancy.

It wasn't until much later that I was able to wrap my head around the complex and deeply sad nature of his suicide. Having been to the brink with my own mental health, I realised how lucky I was to be alive. My medication saved me; he was prescribed some, but it didn't have the chance to kick in. My team saved me; had I not been designated as 'high-risk' and put on suicide watch, I wouldn't have survived my darkest low. I felt angry that Siôn didn't receive the help he needed, and guilty that I did. As is often the case with suicide, I will always wonder, *Could I have done more to help? What if things had been different? Would he still be here?*

I also know how all-encompassing those thoughts can be, and how swift that spiral is. I know that the deepest depression can convince you, with so much clarity, that ending your life is the best option for everyone involved. It was most terrifying that we didn't see it coming. Siôn seemed like the happiest person in every room. I can relate to a lot of what he went through as someone who has struggled with deep depression, but I can never relate to the experience of being a man in this kind of scenario. Men experience different kinds of pressures to stay silent and avoid receiving help – things I will probably never fully comprehend.

Losing someone you love to suicide changes everything. While you can read about the severity of the death toll, you never expect it to be someone close to you. The quick spiral of Sîon's illness demonstrated the fragility of our lives. No person is stronger or weaker than anyone else in the face of mental illness. It can happen to anyone – even people who seem like human sunbeams. Much of my mental health advocacy has emerged from the intense flames of this loss.

It also forced me to confront my own trauma surrounding my mental health. Sometimes, crying for Siôn would lead to hours rocking back and forth in my bedroom, remembering the stark grey of the hospital wards, the voices that told me to look for God, and the ones that told me to end everything. I increased my contact with my doctors during this time, and upped my medication. It was the first time I admitted to myself that my episode and diagnosis had been profoundly terrifying and traumatic. I finally acknowledged that my bipolar came hand in hand with fear: fear of losing my mind again, of sinking into a depression I can't return from, and of leaving my family behind.

The lows that come with my illness can be quick, erratic and delusional. Siôn had loved his life just a few months earlier. It reminded me that I needed to take my health seriously, and to always accept help when I feel I need it. Now, when I haven't slept for multiple nights in a row, I will always ring a doctor. Since then, I have consistently taken my lows seriously.

In the short term, dealing with grief simply comes down to fight-or-flight. It's all about survival and putting one foot in front of the other (and, in my case, dealing with an unexpected high). The long term, though, can be even more complicated and confusing. On one hand, this loss made my fears even deeper. It reminded me that nothing in life is certain; the best things can be snatched away from you at any moment. Years later, this would manifest in my relationship with my boyfriend, when his phone died one evening and I couldn't get hold of him. I spiralled into a panic attack and convinced myself that he had died on the way home. I could no longer tell myself 'that wouldn't happen to me', because it could, and it had.

At the same time, trauma can remind you that most things in life really aren't that bad. Lucy put it best when she said that when the worst thing imaginable happens, everything else feels easier to handle. Everything falls into perspective after a big trauma; whether work is tough, you fall out with a friend, or the guy you're dating stops replying. I watch my colleagues become extremely stressed by presentations or meetings, and I feel almost immune to it. These moments come and go as quickly as they arrive. They're all manageable and solvable.

That isn't to downplay the difficulties we all feel on a daily basis. It's just a reminder of how resilient the human spirit is. In those early weeks, it seemed like Lucy would never emerge from the pain – but time really is a healer. Watching her set up a foundation in Sîon's name, and eventually finding love with someone new, has made me extremely proud. We became very close for the first time in the aftermath of Sîon's death – and we still talk every day now. I realised that our bond is deeper than our childhood bickering had had me believe. My family has been through so much together, and each heartbreak only makes us love one another more.

Sîon still lives on in all of us. After he died, his family coined the term 'Celebrasiôn' as a way to remember the energy and positivity he contributed to everything he did. His depression existed in the shadows, but we will always remember him for the light.

9
finding my voice

After Siôn's passing, and amidst the rollercoaster of changing lockdown restrictions, I felt more motivated than ever to learn about mental health. I knew how it felt to not understand your own mind, to feel incredibly lonely and to believe you're the only person who has ever felt so low. I knew that the more serious aspects of mental health – from psychosis to suicide – were often spoken about in hushed voices. I wanted to change that.

When I was diagnosed with bipolar 1 two years earlier, I still knew so little about my illness. Of course, I received information and support from my medical team, but I desperately wanted to find other people like me – people I could relate to. I wanted to read hopeful stories that would make me feel better about my future. Sadly, my depression-addled attention span didn't allow for any extensive reading or watching, so I turned to online forums for guidance about my illness. This was unhelpful, to say the least.

People say you should never look up your symptoms on Google – and they are right. You hope for a hit of reassurance, but all you get is doom and gloom. I read pages and pages of people complaining about medicines that didn't work or had horrendous side effects, and read tale after tale of repeated manic episodes and suicide attempts. The more awful stories I read, the more I searched for something good to balance them out – and the cycle just continued to worsen.

I understand that there are plenty of people happily living with and managing bipolar 1 – but they tend not to be the ones holed up in online forums. Still, these negative stories made me feel even more hopeless and lost, at a time when I would have given anything for the promise that things would get better.

During that time, my parents frequently mentioned the actor and broadcaster Stephen Fry. He was one of the few celebrities who had been open about his bipolar diagnosis. In the hope of supporting me during those dark months during 2018, my parents ordered a DVD of his documentary, *Stephen Fry: The Secret Life of a Manic Depressive*.

When the DVD eventually arrived (we had ordered it from the USA), my mum and I sat down in the sitting room to watch it with a cup of tea. After thirty minutes, tears were streaming down my face. One scene depicted a man marching around a graveyard, explaining that he speaks to angels every year. All I could think was, *Will that be me? Will I be speaking to my demons throughout my life?* I envisioned myself walking the graveyard of our local church in Gloucestershire – singing 'Angels' by Robbie Williams into the sky. God only knew what my future would look like. It was petrifying.

I know that Stephen Fry is a fantastic role model, and I am sure his open discussions about bipolar have been incredibly helpful for so many. But he was not the role model I was looking for or needed as a 22-year-old girl. It was like being stuck in a six-hour conversation with your dad's friend at a party. You have nothing in common and, to be honest, no matter how nice he is, no one wants to talk to their dad's friend all night. We may both have bipolar, but this is where our similarities end. I wanted to find someone like me – a woman, preferably. Young? Even better. Besides the depressing online forums, I was unsure if these people even existed.

A few months later, the rapper Kanye West dropped his album, *Ye*. The album cover's art was adorned with the words, 'I hate being Bi-Polar it's awesome.' Again, not the kind of role model I was looking for, but I could see myself reflected in Kanye's experiences. I have to admit, this album is one I return to again and again. I couldn't agree more with those words on the cover: they sum up exactly how it feels to have bipolar. On a low day, you hate it, how unfair it feels and how painful it can be. Then when you're up, you get to experience the richest human experience possible. It *does* feel awesome when you're flying high. I think if I released my own album about bipolar, I would call it something similar. Think, *Woohoo! Fuck my life!*

On a more serious note, Kanye's experience of bipolar was, and continues to be, a massive trigger for me. On the one hand, I respect his art and his talent as a musician (to be frank, it makes me want to stop taking my medicines). When people call him a 'genius', I jump to the conclusion that I too would be a genius if I stopped taking my meds. However, on the flip side, I have winced watching his erratic, problematic behaviour unfold, especially the racism, anti-Semitism and public outbursts on social media. His delusions make him seem incredibly unhinged, and just generally a bad person, which I can't help but worry reflects on those of us living with the same condition.

It's complicated. I relate to him in many ways, even though he is extremely rich, famous and talented. When he drops music without warning, or overshares when he feels high, I can relate to that feeling of unstoppable creativity. My bipolar also makes me want to act in ways I'm not proud of. I would *love* to run for president on a high day (although I would never admit that to my friends). Still, seeing the repercussions of Kanye's actions has been useful. I never want to ruin my reputation and my relationships by chasing the delusional thoughts in my mind. I want to exist in the same world as everyone else, even if that's at the expense of being a 'genius'.

Another bipolar character I came across in the aftermath of my diagnosis was the fictional character Carrie, played by Claire Danes in the American drama series *Homeland*. The show first aired in 2011, but I hadn't watched it yet, so I binged all seasons of this with Lucy during lockdown, around the time I was hoping to reduce my medication. I was on a combination of quetiapine (the miracle anti-psychotic) and lithium to stabilise my mood.

Watching Carrie's relationship with her medicines play out in the drama, I felt stressed. Less medication meant she would get on a roll, hunting down terrorists and generally being a bit of a superwoman. But then the tipping point would always involve her losing her mind and not being able to function. I thought, *Is this my trade-off? If I want to live up to my full potential, will I have to fall down the rabbit hole?*

I felt upset at the scenes in which she flushed her pills away, looking in the mirror with the confidence that she could manage her bipolar herself. But she never could – it always took a full hold on her and ended in a breakdown. All I wanted was a normal life, and this show's portrayal of bipolar made me question if that would ever be possible.

I don't think I began to feel hopeful and reassured about bipolar until I started reading mental health memoirs. The first one I read, over Christmas in 2020, was titled *Manic: A Memoir*. Written by Terri Cheney, it was the first extensive, real-life story from a woman I had come across. At first, I felt terrified reading the sensationalist subtitle: *A woman in pain. A life in chaos. The courage to fight a secret madness*. Oh, God! Pain, chaos and madness. I wasn't sure that sounded fun. The book itself wasn't much better. I nearly gave up after reading, in detail, about her suicide attempt, and about how much her bipolar had ruined her relationships and career throughout her life.

While I read her story, it made me feel stiff as a piece of wood, but at the same time I was engrossed. I became hyper-focused, keen to absorb every element of her story. To be fair to Terri, the book ended on a much more reassuring note, about how her diagnosis ultimately saved her life. So maybe everything would be alright for me, too?

My friend told me to watch an episode of the series *Modern Love*, based on Terri's essay, which starred Anne Hathaway in the leading role. I was terrified to watch it – worried that it would be yet another depiction of bipolar that would make me feel hopeless. Instead, it made me feel seen and understood. The way Anne's character described her bipolar, her honesty, her fears ... I could relate to all of it. I felt so grateful for the way she embodied that role and no doubt made so many more people aware of what bipolar disorder actually was.

I thought, *I wish I had seen this when I was first diagnosed. Maybe it wouldn't have been so lonely.*

From that point onwards, I became fixated on absorbing as many accounts of bipolar as I could. I searched 'books about bipolar' and, I won't lie, there weren't many. But I ordered the best ones I could find, and three dropped through my letterbox the next day: *An Unquiet Mind* by Kay Redfield Jamison, *Madness* by Marya Hornbacher and *Living at the Speed of Light* by Kai Conibear. I whizzed through all of these at record speed. It's wild to think I was only really starting my bipolar education, two years after my diagnosis. I was finally learning from women who had made it through the worst of their illness and could share their tools for how to manage it. It felt as if I had opened up a whole new world. *Bipolar disorder exists beyond hospital wards and online forums!* It was a revelation.

The biggest takeaway from all of these books is just how unique each experience of bipolar is. Each book, and each author, is so different; it shows that you can't assume there is only one definitive story of mental illness. There is space for *so* many more. I had only really spoken about bipolar to my close friends and at my Viva Fever events, which would normally leave me with a severe vulnerability hangover.

Speaking about it so publicly scared me to death. This was partly because I still felt that I was in the trenches, learning to navigate my illness with mixed results. I thought: *How can I offer anything useful, when I barely have a handle on this thing myself?* The other part of me was ashamed. I remembered how much I had posted online during my manic episode, and I didn't want to appear to be attention-seeking by speaking about my condition. To this day, I have a strong fear of being disbelieved and misunderstood. I didn't want to open myself up to criticism, when I was already so sensitive. That said, I knew I wanted to contribute in some kind of meaningful way. I just didn't know how.

During lockdown, some friends of friends reached out to ask if I would like to come onto their new podcast about mental health, to talk about my experience with bipolar 1. I said yes, even though I was terrified. I still didn't feel equipped to talk about bipolar. I was still processing the trauma of hospital and beginning to understand my triggers. Sitting in my dad's office at his desk, waiting for the podcast hosts to log onto the Zoom call, my heart was beating hard in my chest.

Is this the right thing to do? I thought.

Instantly, the hosts made me feel at ease, and we chatted about the weather and running before getting into the questions they had prepared. Recording the rest of the show was a blur, but I remember shaking as I answered all their questions. I tried my best to project an air of confidence about my diagnosis, which was quite far away from how I actually felt. In reality, if someone had come up to me and offered to take away my bipolar, I would have instantly said yes, no questions asked. Instead, I tried to keep things light-hearted, finding the funnier moments in my story in a bid to make listeners laugh. I wasn't being purposely disingenuous – it was a bit of 'fake it 'til you make it'. I hoped that one day I would be the bipolar role model I had been craving.

The morning the podcast aired, I went on a long run to listen to it. I felt adrenaline racing through my body, as I couldn't help thinking about all the people who might listen: my old colleagues, my ex, his family. *Will they think I'm attention-seeking? Will they think I'm crazy? Have I done the wrong thing? Should I be hiding this?* The self-hatred and doubt sunk in, and when I got back from my run my tears mingled in with the hot water from the shower.

The actual response from the podcast was a massive surprise. By the time I got dressed, my phone had started blowing up with kind messages about the interview. Some were from people I knew, who didn't know exactly what I had been through. Others were from complete strangers, often people who had bipolar too. Around lunch, I received a DM from a girl who was a similar age to me. She sent me three hefty paragraphs, telling me that her friend had sent her the podcast, and how similar her recent episode had been to mine.

'This gave me hope!' she wrote.

Reading those four words, my fear dissipated. If I could reach even one person with bipolar, it was worth doing. I knew how it felt to be desperate for hope.

I wanted to do more, but it wasn't until the start of 2022 that I had a brain wave about where to go next. My friends planned a trip to Mexico for New Year's Eve in 2021 and I decided to go with them, even though it felt like a gamble. I had been reasonably stable for a full year, without any signs that I might slip into mania again, so that was reassuring. However, I remained in a constant state of low energy, and my binge eating was still out of hand, to the point that I was diagnosed with binge eating disorder. The thought of a holiday scared me, because I constantly felt disgusted with myself. I'd have out-of-control moments of overeating, followed by a day of restriction afterwards. It was far from healthy, and I was worried about being around friends, so far from home, while I was still stuck in this unhealthy cycle.

I had suspected for some time that the lithium I was still on, alongside quetiapine, was the cause of my binge eating. I also knew that in preventing my lows, it was also preventing my highs. I had spoken to my doctors about this, but they always seemed wary about reducing my dose or taking me off it altogether. After all, it's known to be an effective treatment for bipolar, and they wanted me to stay on an even keel. But in the week leading up to my trip away, I decided to trust my gut and stopped taking lithium. Every night, I swallowed only my quetiapine and hoped for the best.

As a warning, I don't recommend this approach. You should always consult a doctor about reducing your medication, and you should always do it slowly. Do as I say, not as I do! My experience with coming off lithium taught me that I could trust my gut, especially when it came to my treatment. If you feel your gut might be telling you something, raise your concerns with your doctor (always do this before making any changes). It's important to remember that what works for others may not work for you.

Within a few days of arriving in Mexico, something felt dramatically different, as if a weight had been lifted off my shoulders. I noticed smells in the air and felt huge waves of gratitude for this beautiful place, for my friends, for my life. Free from lithium and jet-lagged after a long flight, I entered into a hypomanic state for the first time since my episode. I laughed non-stop on that holiday, ran every morning and danced into the early hours with my friends. It was the first time, since hospital, that I wasn't the first person to slope off to bed. I wanted to drink margaritas, chat endlessly and wake up early. My eating habits seemed to resume a normal cycle; I savoured every tortilla chip and taco, but I stopped overeating – and as a result, I stopped *worrying* about overeating. It was pure bliss.

I had been away a few times since my episode, but this was the first time I felt pure joy sinking into my skin alongside the vitamin D. Safe in the knowledge that my quetiapine was keeping full-blown mania at bay, I felt free to enjoy the benefits of the hypomanic state. The rush of adrenaline in the morning, the intense feelings of love, the unreal quality of music in my ears ... I had missed it all so much. I realised that I *wanted* these feelings. I didn't want to suppress them. They made me feel like myself. Yes, they are bipolar – but they are also mine.

The end of the holiday wasn't quite so positive, though. After accidentally drinking water from the shower that seemed to be contaminated, I was one of four people on the trip throwing up during the last few days and on the plane journey home (would not recommend). What I didn't realise was that in throwing up my entire guts, I had also removed my miracle anti-psychotic from my system. This gap, just a few days with not one single bit of medicine in my body, exposed me to the most dangerous hypomanic state I had been in since September 2018.

That week, jet-lagged and under-medicated, I experienced epiphany after epiphany.

> *I NEED TO BUILD VIVA FEVER!*
> *I'M SO HAPPY, I WANT TO MEET OTHER*
> *PEOPLE WITH THIS SO I CAN HELP THEM!*
> *I WANT TO CHANGE THE WORLD!*
> *I WANT TO MAKE A DIFFERENCE!*
> *I WANT TO TELL MY STORY ... NOT JUST TO*
> *A COMMUNITY, BUT TO THE WORLD!!!*

One night, at around 4 a.m. when I couldn't sleep, I decided there was only one thing for it – I needed to make a documentary. Just like Stephen Fry's, except presented by a young female: me. *Surely the world needed this? Surely this would help me reach young women who had been through what I've been through?*

The idea of presenting my own documentary wasn't completely out of the ordinary. Back in 2018 – the year of my depressive, anxious spiral into eventual madness – I actually started making some showreels with a friend who was a photographer and videographer. It seems strange that I would pursue this line of work while I was in such a bad state, but something about speaking in front of the camera seemed to calm me – at least, it did eventually after a few very stiff takes. It felt like an extension of modelling but with some added freedom and expression. Interviewing random people outside a Beyoncé concert was so much fun and lifted my mood immediately. In my bones, I felt this was something I was good at, and that I could become even better.

Later, once I left the hospital, I rewatched these videos and wondered if I could ever get back there. This part of me had been lying dormant for such a long time. So when the brain wave appeared to make a documentary, it genuinely felt like destiny.

Hours later, I phoned an acquaintance who was starting out in directing (let's call him J) and asked if I could meet him the following day.

Maybe he will know how I can make a world-changing documentary and open up the conversation amongst young people?

He agreed, and I took this as a sign from the universe (or God, perhaps) that everything would fall into place.

On a beautiful cold, sunny January morning, I arrived at the director's house, having run 10 km before 8 a.m., armed with a bag of croissants that cost £25. At this point, I had been saving my modelling money for years to buy a flat. My racing thoughts told me that I was rich, life was perfect, and this was day one of making a documentary that would go down in history as one of the most influential, groundbreaking portrayals of mental health – OF ALL TIME! Spending £25 on croissants seemed like a completely reasonable use of money. I was celebrating, after all.

I sat opposite J and spoke at 1,000 mph about my idea, all while holding a small digital camera, which I somehow thought was all I needed. My grandiose thoughts must have been pretty convincing, because he said he would love to make the documentary with me – as long as I could fund it.

Looking back on this moment, I feel extremely sad. I don't think either of us realised, at that point, just how vulnerable I was, especially when it came to spending. I talked confidently about how much money I had. I was elated and not necessarily being realistic. On a normal day, perhaps I would have discovered how these things usually come about. You would meet a production company, which would then pitch to a TV channel to fund the project. I was too excited to dig any deeper, so I agreed to start the process myself, entirely self-funded.

Within a week, J had found a DOP/videographer to work with us on the project, and we spent lots of time together plotting out how the documentary should look. And then we got to work. We put out call-outs on social media and reached out to charities including Bipolar UK. Between the three of us, we secured five interviews with people diagnosed with bipolar 1 for me to interview on camera. I was so excited to meet other people who were just like me and hopefully learn from them.

Although the intensity of my post-Mexico hypomania subsided, and my quetiapine kicked into gear, I was still undeniably high throughout the whole experience of filming the documentary. It was the most creatively stimulating thing I had ever done, and I bounced home from my meetings and interviews feeling more alive than ever. Meeting other young people with bipolar was absolute magic. We were strangers, but we understood each other so deeply. In the interviews, we exchanged stories about mania, laughed at the highs and experienced a sense of profound understanding and empathy when discussing the lows. I knew I had made friends for life in the process of making this documentary.

On top of that, we reached out to medical professionals. I couldn't believe how freeing it was to speak to professionals outside a patient-doctor situation. I suddenly felt more confident to ask 'silly' questions such as, 'Can coffee be a trigger?' (Yes, it turns out, and it's a biggie for me!)

Alongside all of this, I loved being on set, talking about camera angles and seeing our short film come to life. I felt as if I had whizzed back in time to that wide-eyed model in New York, wandering around the city with a photographer's eye. I truly believed the footage we were recording was gold dust, and I couldn't wait for the world to see it.

Sadly, that footage would never see the light of day and the disk remains on my shelf, covered in dust. I should have known that my shiny carefree attitude would eventually come crashing down.

After we had shot everything, J arranged for the footage to be sent to an editor who could knock it all into shape. For three weeks, I locked myself away to view everything, taking notes on every second of each interview, writing down my thoughts about how the film should run. I printed it out and handed it to the editor. I can imagine she was quite taken aback by my pages and pages of notes and ideas. It wasn't exactly 'normal' to have extensive notes on every minute of footage – but I couldn't help it. I was so excited about this project I had poured my heart into, and I couldn't wait to see everything come together.

Not long after, I sensed something wasn't right. J prevented me from emailing the editor directly, and I felt that I was being left out of discussions. I had spent £7,000 of my own money on this project so far, and I wasn't trusted to be a part of the editing conversation.

Why is he treating me like a child? I thought.

This dynamic went on for months, until eventually I became so frustrated that I marched into the editor's office and asked for her email address so I could contact her myself. After I left, I sent a long message explaining that I wanted to be involved in the editing discussions, given it was such a sensitive topic for me. When I emerged from the Tube on the other side of my journey, I had ten missed calls from J. I picked up his latest call and was met by a scream down the phone.

'This is a professional relationship I have, and you're ruining it, Rosie!' he shouted. 'You are impulsive and impossible to work with!'

My heart sank. I immediately felt embarrassed and physically sick. This project was supposed to help me demystify bipolar and discredit some of the assumptions made about the condition. And yet, the man I had trusted to tell my story accused me of being the very stereotype that people with bipolar receive all the time. *Impossible. Impulsive.* My high well and truly disintegrated. I could feel my mind tumbling back down, down, down.

After I hung up the phone with J, I went straight back home and got into bed. And so began my longest-lasting low since I had left the hospital. This led me to extend my care and increase my medicine dose. I received several messages from J over the coming weeks, each one harsher than the last, as the project inevitably fell apart. Every upbeat thought I had about bipolar fell into the deep blue, as I sunk into suicidal ideation and believed everyone found me impossible to be around. I couldn't get out of bed, I couldn't run, and the shame of spending £7,000 on an unfinished project engulfed me. I have never felt as bipolar as I did in those months of working on that documentary. The high was incredible, and I had never felt so inspired. But the depression that followed was unbearable.

The silver lining? The people I met in the process. Some of the young people I interviewed about their experiences with bipolar ended up becoming close friends. They checked in on me, and they helped me rebuild my confidence again to pursue making a documentary.

'Don't give up,' they told me. 'Our voices matter – and your voice matters.'

As I slowly emerged from my depressive state (what goes down must come up again, after all), I noticed a follower on my Instagram page – Sam, who was a producer at Channel 4. Impulsive Rosie came out again, and I decided to drop him a DM to ask if he would meet me for a coffee.

'I've made a documentary and I don't know what to do with it,' I wrote. 'It's nowhere near being finished … but I know that what I'm looking into is important.'

Sam turned out to be a total legend and made me feel comfortable enough to tell him everything that had happened: the hypomania, the expensive footage I had no idea how to finish, the breakdown in my relationship with the former director, and the panic attacks that ensued. Thankfully, the editor I worked with before had cut a 'sizzle' for me out of our footage – essentially, a little trailer that gives a sense of the vibe. I handed Sam my headphones to watch it right there in the café. I could see his eyes light up, and he promised me that he would try to find a way to fund the rest of my documentary and get it onto Channel 4.

Several months passed before anything happened. Sam checked in sporadically, telling me he hadn't forgotten about me and was still working on it behind the scenes. In the meantime, my life felt pretty unstable. I was adjusting to the extreme moods that being on only one medicine – quetiapine – could bring. The highs were high, but, my God, the lows were low. I would have hypomania one week, waking up early, drinking endless coffees, spending excessive amounts of money (including on my flat in East London, which was probably the one wise monetary choice during this time).

During these episodes, I would share ten stories on my Instagram every day, documenting my epiphanies. But before long, I would crash, delete everything, cancel on friends and feel unable to go into work. I was still modelling, but not enough to feel confident about my job. My fluctuations were so intense that I was terrified I would never be able to manage without constant medical support. My mind swam with existential questions (yes, even more than the usual twenty-five-year-old's). *Should I go back on lithium? What job should I do? Will this ever become easier to deal with?*

And then, on a summer's day in 2022, Sam called me out of the blue. 'I've found a way to get this on Channel 4,' he said. 'It will have to be a new documentary though. You'll be starting again with a new production company – but don't worry, you won't regret this.'

When I hung up the phone, I burst into tears. This was the best outcome I could have hoped for. I didn't want everything I had already done to go to waste, but I also needed a fresh start. That week, I met with my new director (a woman, this time) over Zoom. I felt so calm with her and ready to open up and pour my heart out again on this project. I was still terrified, but I kept thinking about how much it would have helped me to see a documentary about bipolar on Channel 4. It would have made the future feel less weird and unknown.

Filming for 'Modelling, Mania and Me' started only a few months later. Julia, the director, was very keen to capture me as Real Rosie, rather than Performer Rosie who always wanted to make light of things. She asked me to film my mood swings whenever they came for snippets in the documentary. The first time I recorded myself during a mood swing, my negative thoughts told me that filming myself crying was attention-seeking and inappropriate. But Julia told me that this content was valuable, and it became much easier. Soon, I was accustomed to whipping out my phone whenever I felt a low or high coming on. I noticed just how frequently and dramatically my moods flipped, and how obvious the diagnosis was in my everyday life.

While we were filming, I had no idea how the documentary would be received. I just knew that I trusted Julia to capture me and my bipolar in a way that wasn't sensationalised or trying to create a narrative that wasn't there. Then, after six months of filming, she arrived at my house to show me the first cut of the documentary. As I watched those twenty minutes of footage, I couldn't help tearing up. The narrative followed me through falling in love (more on that in the next chapter), pushing past anxieties, and getting the subject of bipolar into *Women's Health* magazine.

I was surprised by how quickly the documentary aired. It was posted on Channel 4's YouTube channel, and I went onto radio shows and TV to talk about it in the run-up to its release. I had become so much more confident since my first podcast. I knew that bipolar wouldn't ever be in the rearview mirror, but that was OK. I had made peace (as far as I could) with the highs and lows. It felt good to talk about it.

Bipolar UK held a screening to mark the documentary's release, which was so wonderful and overwhelming, having all my favourite people come out to support me. The next day, my sister messaged me to say that the documentary had hit 10,000 views. I couldn't believe it! And then it kept doubling, and doubling, until it reached 100,000 views within the first month. While I know that reading the comments section is usually risky business, I found so much comfort in reading people's responses. There were so many people commenting about how much my story reflected theirs.

I'm so proud of everything that came out of that project. I feel relieved that it is now out in the world for anyone to find, so that other people might feel seen and understood. We're not alone in the chaos of our minds, even though it feels like the loneliest place on the planet. Proudly speaking up about my bipolar has taught me that.

I would love to say that it's now easier to speak openly about my experiences, but I think it will always feel a bit uncomfortable. That nagging voice is always there, telling me that if I continually talk about bipolar, it will be the only thing that defines me. *Everyone has already heard this, Rosie! No one cares anymore!* But with each lovely message I receive, I'm reminded that it *is* worthwhile.

That loveliness spurs me on – but so does the confusion. I have noticed that when I speak about bipolar, some people have no idea what to say. There have been times when I have mentioned my bipolar or suicide ideation or psychosis, and the energy in the room has completely drained.

I get it, of course, but it's a reminder that we need to demystify these serious aspects of mental health. The more we all know, the more we can spot the signs in the people we love and in ourselves. Knowledge is power. It's the only way we can break the stigma.

That's not to say everyone who has ever experienced mental ill-health should speak publicly about their experiences. You don't owe anyone anything. I understand why you would want to just get on with your life, especially when times are good. When your brain feels abnormal, it can feel like a blessing to live life normally and not talk about what you've been through. I completely respect that. My world has opened up since I've been more open about bipolar, but that's not the journey for everyone. It's your process, and don't let anyone tell you otherwise. We all have to find our own ways to cope.

That said, if you *do* want to share more, but you're just not sure how, I recommend starting with the people you really trust. Open up about a part of your mental health that you wouldn't normally speak about. For example, what it feels like to be high. I used to go bright red if I spoke about the extent of my high thoughts with my friends – how highly I think of myself, and how religious I become (*Will they think I'm crazy?*) – but they were so interested and engaged, which meant they were better able to understand and support me during a high. This then gave me the courage to open up outside my close circles. It helped me to remove some of the shame I experience about having bipolar. I have surrendered to the fact that there will always be people who don't understand. It's the people who *try* to understand that really count.

I'm pleased to say representations of bipolar seem to have come a long way since I first started looking. From the BBC comedy, *Big Mood*, that aired last year, to this very book you're holding in your hands, young bipolar voices are becoming more prominent. I still struggle to relate to every experience, and perhaps you will struggle to relate to me. But I have realised that, as much as we can find comfort in other's experiences, we all have our own unique experiences with mental health. You have to stay focused on your own road. It's possible for two things to be true at the same time: you're on your own path, but you're also never alone.

10
loving (and losing) with bipolar

One of the things I struggle with most is how bipolar impacts my 'normal' human emotions, particularly love. Do I get so swept up in love because I'm bipolar? Is it normal to feel *so* much? What even *is* normal when it comes to love? Getting obsessed with boys, pining over exes, sending regrettable texts in the middle of the night ... isn't that what every twenty-something does? Or is it just another sign that my mind works in extremes?

To understand this better, we need to rewind to before I received my diagnosis. I have always loved the idea of love, and you could say I was a boy-obsessed teenager. But that's par for the course for young girls. I grew up on a diet of romcoms, and magazines that included posters of fit topless pop stars that you could rip out and plaster on your wall. I was also privileged to grow up in a home with parents who met in their early twenties and had an amazing relationship. Even today, in their seventies, they adore each other. This was the example I was given: love is destined, it comes easy, and it lasts forever.

With that in mind, I fell head over heels for a boy who resembled Justin Bieber on my first day of senior school. He even played the guitar and sang at school events – swoon! I 'got with him' at our first school social, while Katy B's 'On a Mission' swept through the dance floor. Having had a few clandestine swigs of Malibu, I truly believed this boy was the love of my life. However, Bieber 2.0 had other plans and quickly found himself a very cool, model girlfriend.

I was only fifteen at the time, but my reaction to this news was pretty extreme, given I hardly knew the boy. The day I found out, I cried the whole way home in the car and sobbed for the entire evening in my room. For weeks, I isolated myself, scribbling furiously in my diary, and going for long, moody walks listening to indie music on my iPod. I knew I was depressed, but I was too young to have the language to describe how I felt. As we know, I became hyper-focused on becoming a model to outshine this girl and win my indie heartthrob back (it was very *Legally Blonde* of me).

Suffice to say, it didn't work out. Just like Elle Woods, I realised that the boy wasn't worth it but the career actually was. In my later teenage years, I lost all desire to pursue boys. As I have said, I was extremely depressed at this time (which led to my hypothyroidism diagnosis) and I spent my holidays trying to pursue modelling, so love was the last thing on my mind. But once I left school and started working in Abercrombie (cringe) in London, I found a new obsession.

I must have been on my second or third shift when a boy came up to me in the stockroom and asked for my number. He was working part-time but was actually a pianist and West End actor (I'm a sucker for performers).

The night of our first date, he took me to several sticky bars around Piccadilly Circus, where we kicked back sweet cocktails and talked endlessly about music and life. Retracing my steps, I now realise that he took me on a whistle-stop tour past all the life-sized posters of him in his West End show. A red flag, I'd say now, but I was far too excited to notice.

After kissing on the pavement (near his poster) and bouncing home, I wrote in my diary that I had never been happier and that life was perfect. Judging by this entry, I had flown into a hypomanic state, and I stopped sleeping for a week before seeing him next. I envisioned him laughing with my parents (they would *love* their new son-in-law); I imagined sitting front row at one of his performances with tears in my eyes; I imagined what our kids would be like.

Long story short, I saw on social media after two more dates that he was back with his ex. And so, the intense heartbreak came. I cried for days, got into bed every day at 6 p.m., cancelled all my shifts and obsessed over pictures of his girlfriend on Facebook. The pain lasted for months. Again, I wrote endless diary entries, swearing and ranting about how much I hated him. I think I knew, even then, that my anger was irrational – but still, I was furious that he had stolen away my imagined future and ruined my life. Six months after our 'break-up', my sister Amii insisted that we watch him in his West End musical. As she predicted, this taught me the meaning of getting the 'ick'.

I emerged from my heartbreak hole but was acutely aware that six months of depression and anger after a three-date relationship was *not cool* and most certainly not normal. I became terrified to date again. The connection between boys and depression felt impossible to ignore. And so, as my career took me to Paris, New York and Berlin,

I stayed away from dating and relationships, terrified of the chaos they could bring.

It wasn't until I met B in 2017 that opening myself up again felt worth the risk. It's hard to say whether our relationship felt so perfect in those early months because of hypomania, or because it actually was. Each morning, I woke up and felt excited for our conversations. After every social event, we would leave holding hands and debrief on the way home. We sent each other songs all day and then listened together at night. When he walked into the room, I felt unable to concentrate. He brought out my weirdest sense of humour, and we formed a new language that only we could speak. It was young love, my first proper relationship, and the honeymoon period.

You already know about my spiral into depression, the deterioration of our relationship, and the break-up that sent me into mania – so I won't repeat the details for both of our sakes. But what I haven't mentioned is how that mania inevitably delayed the 'processing' part of that break-up. For one, I was completely away with the fairies for months, so I couldn't even think about what had happened, let alone work through those emotions. And then I transferred my obsession from B onto my nurse, K, and you know how that worked out (terribly). So, my unprocessed heartbreak lingered over everything throughout my recovery.

B had, understandably, been very worried when I was admitted to hospital. In the months that followed, he checked in every once in a while to see how I was. In low moments, my mind repeatedly told me how embarrassing I had been.

> *People say they go 'psychotic' after a break-up for dramatic effect, but you literally went psychotic.*
> *You're absolutely pathetic.*

His life was going from strength to strength, while mine was dominated by my illness. His success was just another reminder of the desperate state my life had become, and everything I had lost. I used to be a bright shiny star, too – but those days were over. I missed him and couldn't help replaying the memories of our blissful time together. Maybe it had been magnified because of hypomania, but it was *real love*. Wasn't it? How would I ever find something so pure and true again?

In high moments, though, my mind told me that he was still in love with me and desperate for us to get back together. I wrote him a few questionable letters, and even invited him on holiday with my friends at one point. My mind convinced me that he was my destiny, that my manic episode had been a sign we never should have broken up. The day after sending texts or impulsive letters in the post, reality would hit me. It was over and had been for years. He had moved on. I needed to as well. The regret was crushing.

As I began to come to terms with my bipolar, I felt even more sure that my mind was a dark cloud that would hang over every relationship. I was scared to put myself in the position to love again, knowing where it would inevitably lead. I decided that lifelong singledom was my destiny. All that being said, I still thought it was a great idea to date as much as possible.

While I was living with Moya, working my way through a series of fruitless jobs, dating seemed to be one aspect of my life I could control. It gave me a feeling of normalcy. I hoped my dating escapades would also give me something to talk about, given my career was a touchy subject, and I wanted to avoid talking about my mental health at all costs.

I'm a 23-year-old girl living in London! Yeah, I have the dating apps! Yeah, I go on dates! No, there's nothing wrong with me! Everything's totally normal and completely fine!

If I'm being really honest, I didn't believe the lie I had told myself – that I was destined for singleness forever. The temptation to fall for someone again still felt strong. From all the people I have spoken to with bipolar, I've noticed that love is a huge priority, no matter how much pain it can bring, and no matter how risky it is. The depth, the richness of those emotions, the extreme moods we experience around it … it can be addictive, to say the least.

I have always had an addictive personality. Most of my addictions have been niche and mostly edible, such as Robinsons squash, lollipops and peanut butter (still an issue). Second only to nicotine, dating apps must have been the most annoying addiction I've ever had. While I still found it very difficult to concentrate, I noticed the hours would fly by when I was scrolling through the apps, puffing away at my vape. I was intrigued by just how little I found people attractive.

Vanity ick-ed me out, and I think in this lonely time it was almost a way of hurting myself to scroll through this sea of men and think, *There is no one out there for me.* But then, every so often, I would come across someone who looked like a good egg. Minimal pictures, smiley face, kind eyes. I kept on scrolling because I was hunting for hope. And then it would come – a hit of dopamine.

Still, even going on constant dates, I felt numb. I'm sure the lithium had something to do with it. My sex drive was almost non-existent, and I felt distant from pretty much everyone I met. Sometimes I told the men I dated about my bipolar; sometimes I didn't. I noticed that when I did, I would overshare and try to make out I had absolutely everything under control. I would imply that I was someone who only got the highs, barely the lows, to come across as fun and take the edge off a serious conversation.

The reality at that time, if I'm honest, was that I still had no idea how to manage really. I was lying to cover up something most people didn't know anything about or found quite worrying. It wasn't until the end of 2020, when I decided to come off my lithium and my highs well and truly returned, that the thrill of romance properly came back.

It started when I swiped past a really fit man on one of the apps. He looked a lot like my ex (red flag), except he was covered in tattoos. But there was one problem: I quickly realised that the dating profile was not in fact the man I fancied but was his friend. So, I did what every normal (?!) person would do and tracked down this fit friend; first by looking up the guy on Instagram, and then scrolling until I found the friend. One night, under the influence of alcohol that was fuelling the high, I decided to DM Tattoo Man to find out if he was single. Very quickly, he replied saying, 'I have a girlfriend, but I'd go on a date if I didn't' (red flag number 2).

Instead of taking this crucial information that he wasn't available, my bipolar thoughts flew out as I explained to him that we were destined to be together in the end. Can we just take a second to imagine receiving this message from a random person – would you reply? I probably wouldn't, but this man continued to engage with my delusions. In my high state of mind, I thought I was the funniest person on the planet, so I asked him to guess which curry I had ordered, sending laughing emojis as though this was a really fun game for him. I think he played along because he was intrigued by the absolute chaos I'd dropped into his DMs. I added further fuel to the fire when I watched a video about manifestation that said to lie down for five minutes while envisioning your future. Every day that week, high as a kite, I envisioned him in my mind, believing I had the power to control my future – and that Tattoo Man was in it.

I would love to say it ended there, but I went on to send him sporadic messages during hypomanic episodes over the years. He's still with his girlfriend. I still know basically nothing about him. Utterly embarrassing behaviour.

Next up, there was my dalliance with a man we can call Surfer Boy. I met him at a dinner party. He was from Devon, and the Gloucestershire girl inside me felt drawn to his outdoorsy vibe. He had blond hair and a tan, and looked like a model (old habits die hard). As soon as our eyes locked, I had decided it was love. He seemed equally enamoured with me (at least at first), so we started seeing each other for walks and morning runs. I would send him pictures of me, and he would respond with heart-eye emojis. I snapped a photo of him on my balcony eating a bowl of cereal, and I remember thinking, *He is the fittest man I have ever seen.*

The first time we slept together, I believed he was the love of my life. I thought that I had never met someone so attractive, and I couldn't sleep for a week afterwards because all I could think about was the next time I could see him again. To make matters worse, apart from a brief experience with uncontrollable lust the year before, this was the first time I was absolutely consumed by it. A classic by-product of hypomania, this is known as hypersexuality – I wanted to have sex *all the time*. I had never been a very sexual person.

In fact, in school I was labelled 'Granny' for my prudish tendencies. I assumed that this hypersexual Rosie was simply unsurprising in the face of this outrageously attractive man and the electric sparks between us. I was certain that we shared a deep, undeniable sexual chemistry, and that he didn't want to keep his hands off me either. I was convinced that my body was simply reacting to destiny.

SURFER BOY IS MY DESTINY!!!!

As a result, I acted in ways that make me look back and cringe. My language changed, I couldn't stop speaking in 'dirty talk', and I pushed to see him every night so we could sleep together. At one point, he suggested a weekend away and I blurted out, 'SO WE CAN HAVE LOTS OF SEX.' I couldn't help myself. He knew I had bipolar, but this isn't a commonly known symptom and I didn't even know about it at the time. He picked up on the weirdness of my behaviour and began to pull back. Eventually, he ghosted me, and I was absolutely mortified.

Over the following weeks, I saw him around via our mutual friends, and I went scarlet-red each time. I was sure he had told everyone about my insatiable, obsessive sex drive, and how it became a 'bit much'. The shame pushed me into a low that led me to extend my care. After my psychotic episode, I had been given three years of support. This 'romance' happened around the end of that. With the suicidal ideation, the sudden need to increase all of my medicines, and my depression, I worried that I would never be able to let go of the support.

On top of that, this hypersexual episode couldn't help but make me think, *What else does bipolar make you do?! What other weird symptoms will I find out about?*

I couldn't believe I was discovering new symptoms of my bipolar two years after leaving hospital. What more fresh hell would it bring?

While working on my documentary to show the importance of peer support, I interviewed a woman who had experienced hypersexuality during her time at university. As I listened to her speak, I connected to those feelings of shame. It made me wonder how many people out there had been slut-shamed, or ended up in big trouble, because of this hidden sign of bipolar.

If I'm honest, hypersexuality still scares me. It's forced me to stay away from people I find extremely attractive, because it feels like dangerous territory. I never want to push people away because of a side of myself that I can't connect to.

I made sure I stayed away from that level of attraction when I entered my next relationship. We will call him Ibiza Boy, because I invited him on a group holiday to Ibiza with my friends, only to break up with him two days into the trip (savage). I started dating him because I was trying to push past my usual obsession for creative types and try something new. He was also from the countryside and worked in a city job. As silly as it sounds, we bonded over the fact that we both smoked like chimneys but still loved running. He seemed to do everything in extremes – partying hard and exercising hard – which fit perfectly into my bipolar rhythm. Yet I knew from the get-go that he was not my person. I'm not sure exactly why I thought it was a good idea to invite him to Ibiza on my friends' annual group holiday four months after we met, or why I said 'yes' when he asked me to be his girlfriend on the night that we landed there.

It all unravelled on the second day of that holiday.

After seeing my friend in a bikini earlier that day, he said to me – in the privacy of our room – 'You could get your physique like that if you wanted.'

My mood instantly swung into a deep, dark place. I couldn't even communicate with him – I was so taken aback by his brazen comment. We went to the beach after leaving the room, and I lay on the sand with my head in my hands, listening to music, unable to be anywhere near him. I knew that the only way I could escape this spiral was to ask him to leave.

Later that day, I pulled him aside for a chat by the hot tub (very *Love Island*) and burst out with my speech – that it wasn't the right relationship for me, and I needed him to leave this island at the earliest convenience. I knew he had to go, I needed to be with my friends and get back to my baseline. The fact he had triggered this deep low for twenty-four hours was all the evidence I needed that our relationship would never work.

I could tell by his expression that he thought I was impulsive and irrational. When he said, 'I can't tell if this is you or the bipolar,' this solidified my decision.

When I came back to London, the low continued. I was relieved that this man was out of my life, but he had stripped me of the confidence that had taken so long for me to rebuild. I felt acutely aware of my bipolar, of my extreme impulses and reactions. When I caught my reflection in every café or shop window, that insecure voice returned with: *You're fat and disgusting.* I felt out of control for weeks. I hated men. I hated their impact on me. I hated how they made me feel and act. My mind was already enough of a battle I had to deal with. Relationships only seemed to make that battle ten times worse.

And yet ... the lure of the dating apps was addictive. I couldn't think of anything I wanted to do less than going on a date, but I also wanted a distraction. Soon after Ibiza, I wanted to cover up my body as much as I could, having slipped into bingeing since I had returned. I felt gross and my skin was breaking out, but I matched with a guy who had liked me months earlier and commented on the Keane song that was playing in the background of my profile. Let's call him M.

The timing couldn't have been worse, but something told me to just go on a date anyway. Was it fate? Or just another impulse? We met the following Tuesday. I wore an all-black outfit with a big blazer to hide my body. I saw M bounding across the road with his rucksack on, and I felt instantly comfortable. We sat in a bar and skipped all small talk from the get-go.

He worked in documentaries, so I told him about mine (which meant bipolar featured heavily in our conversation). We connected over our passion for storytelling. I felt so intrigued by him. I was curious about everything he said, what he did for work, and what brought him to be sitting opposite me that evening. Four margaritas later, my body was still stiff from the past few weeks, but I felt a warmth and kindness in him that softened my edges. Getting the bus home together (as we lived in the same neighbourhood), we kissed at the bus stop. I could have sworn time stopped a little. (Cringe, but true.) I was still hurting from the mental scars left by Ibiza Boy, but I somehow knew that this was worth pursuing, no matter how bad the timing was.

On one of our early dates, we went to a festival in West London and held hands and chatted in the centre of the dance floor. Our cab back home took an hour, and we talked the whole time about our complexities and our characters. When we slept together, I didn't feel any sort of hypersexuality. I was genuinely attracted to him, calmer and much more myself. Our next few dates happened in quick succession, and we became inseparable over the following few weeks.

Around that time, I also found out that my documentary had been commissioned by Channel 4. Bipolar is confusing – in the same way bad news can spin me high, good news can send me low. My life made more sense than it ever had – I had achieved something I had been working towards for so long, and I could feel myself falling in love. And yet I couldn't stop crying. Life felt painful but beautiful at the same time. I was moving forward in a lot of ways, but that discomfort scared me.

My mood flipped a lot during that time. I called my mum regularly (even more than usual), as I freaked out again and again. I spoke to M too, explaining my fears, telling him about the ways in which love (and obsession) had sent me to dangerous places in the past. He told me his fears too. He was older than me and wanted to make sure his next serious relationship was 'the one'. We had both put up defensive walls, and we both worked to tear the other's down.

M constantly complimented my character, focused little on my appearance (just what I needed) and was always interested in my family and friends. There was so much respect between us, and over time I dared to believe that I could be happily in love, despite my bipolar. A year after we met, we moved in together. M had just bought the flat, which I had helped him choose. Looking around homes together, it felt that we were building our future.

Bipolar had been a big feature of our relationship right from the start, as M had advised me on my documentary and knew about everything I had been through to get there. He never made it into a big deal; he treated it as a noble extra thing I had to deal with alongside my otherwise exciting twenties. But living with a partner – for the first time ever, and especially for the first time since my diagnosis – could be challenging.

Besides Moya and my parents, very few people had seen the full extent of my highs and lows. I know that it can be difficult to deal with someone who can be so unstable. In a way, there's something very comforting about having privacy when my moods swing so aggressively. I have found that the best thing to do is not pay too much attention to the swings. Having someone else around, where every high and low became a long conversation and late night, turned my moods into the centre of gravity at home. I know M only wanted to help, but it made me paranoid about how much my bipolar was impacting him. I would go from barely being able to speak one day, thanks to crushing depression, to being so high that I would come back from a 10 km run wanting to stay up talking for hours. I could sense that it was giving him whiplash, but I couldn't always control it.

Regardless of bipolar, my relationship with M was always extremely loving and we were very tactile. I would always feel most at ease with my hand on his back in any situation or holding his hand as we walked down our street. M was very open to doing the things I loved when he could, and we bonded heavily over our love of spending time with our families. On a night out, I knew that as soon as I needed to go to bed he would never let me go alone, taking my feelings into account in any situation. Our conversations would always stimulate me, and I felt so invested in his career and his friendships. However, our differences became clearer when we moved in together. While I was excited about our future, I know he was worried about our age gap and our differing interests.

Over Christmas that year, we went home to our respective families, and I sunk into a low as I could feel M pulling away. When we came back to the flat for New Year's Eve, I knew this wasn't just my irrational bipolar brain talking – he had one foot out of the door. He had started double-booking when we had plans. Where he would once hug me in the evening, he now procrastinated, and he stopped asking me questions outside of, 'How was your day?'

We were drifting apart, and I didn't know what to do about it. Every interaction felt so fragile; even just sitting on the sofa watching a movie together, the weight of the decision seemed to hang in the air. The flat no longer felt like my home. It was unsettling. Thankfully, at this time I was training for the London Marathon. Leaving the house for my long runs helped so much. Running always helps me to have positive thoughts and gives me a moment to address my internal dialogue. On one run, on a cold January day, I knew I had to be honest with myself. *Why am I so terrified of losing M? Is it him, or does it come from my fear of break-ups and the spiral that could come afterwards? How would it feel to speak to him about my concerns?*

And so I did.

In many ways, M and I were closer than ever towards the end of our relationship, but in other ways we were worlds apart. Our communication was truthful yet guarded. We broke up one Saturday evening in February. My heartbeat kept me awake for twenty-four hours while the tears kept coming.

There were the usual challenges of a break-up to contend with: moving out, grieving the loss of something I hoped was forever, and missing someone I thought the world of. And then there were the bipolar challenges: the fear of keeping myself on an even keel, overanalysing my moods and worrying if I was processing the break-up in the 'right' way.

The mood swings were sharp and strong. I would smoke a whole pack of cigarettes in a day, laughing with friends and being the life and soul of the party, before crying hysterically when I arrived home. In some moments, I felt relieved; in others, I felt that I had lost everything. And the swinging pendulum made me beat myself up more. *How can I not know how I feel? Why are my moods so confusing? What the hell does a normal break-up look like? Is this it?*

In my low moments, I couldn't help thinking about the role my bipolar played in the breakdown of our relationship. M assured me it didn't, and of course there was much more to the story. My friends reminded me of the issues we had that were completely unrelated to my moods. But the lingering thoughts remained: *You caused this. You're impossible to live with. You're unlovable.*

It's normal to feel grief and self-doubt after a break-up; you second-guess your intuition and your belief that this would work out. But here I took it one step further. I questioned whether all my thoughts were grand. If he really was my person, or if I just thought he was. Whether I was deluded. Was it bipolar? Or was it me?

In high moments, I would message M. *Do you think we should give it another go?!*

I don't think that's a good idea, Rosie. You know it wasn't right, he would respond.

On one occasion, I called my mum, convinced in my conviction that he was desperate to get back with me.

'Rosie, you're being deluded,' she responded – and just like that, I crashed back down to earth.

How could I be aware of my tendency to be deluded, yet still feel completely convinced of a delusion when it arrived? It was (and still is) terrifying, to be reminded of how my bipolar could creep up on me without me noticing.

I know we made the right decision, but I remain grateful for everything that relationship taught me. M was always so patient and kind throughout my mood swings, right until the end. After all the terrible situationships, he restored my faith that I could be in a loving relationship one day.

Although I don't know when I'll feel ready, I'm willing to admit that I want love in my future. Love is one hell of a drug for the bipolar brain, and the incredible highs feel worth all the potential risks. I guess that's the same for everyone, right? Love is always a risk. It can heal you or it can hurt you, and sometimes it'll do both. I know that this can be more extreme for me. The lows might be lower, but my God, the highs are higher, and I choose to view that as a gift.

While romantic love still scares me, I know I have so much love in my life regardless.

There are my incredible parents, who put their lives on hold to help me recover. And, of course, my sisters. We have all been through so much together, from Amii holding me in A&E on the day of my episode, to us holding Lucy after she lost her partner. I'm grateful for this supportive sisterhood – one defined by humour, light and silliness. It was always an unconditional bond, but now it's a friendship bond too.

There are the friends who stuck by me throughout all the chaos and have continued to make me feel loved and accepted – when it would have been so easy to abandon me altogether. My school friends, Rosa, Alicia and

Maddie, constantly checked in to say they were thinking of me, even when I shut them – and everyone – out for months on end.

I will always remember when Rosa came round to my house while I was on suicide watch, and how she held me in her arms in my garden as I cried hysterically. She told me to trust her, that one day we would look back on this day from a position of good health, and we would remember how far I had come. She was right. Training for a half marathon together last October, smiling and laughing the whole way, has definitely been a highlight of the friendship ever since.

I also remember when Maddie invited me to a big dinner at her house for New Year's Eve in 2019 while I was at rock bottom. She understood completely when I crept upstairs to bed at 9 p.m. She came up to cuddle me and made it known that we were still celebrating the New Year together and that there would be many more to come.

Their kindness gave me hope when I thought I had lost all of it.

There are the friends I made in London through modelling, too. I met Sarah when I was sixteen. We had both booked a job on a music video and instantly became inseparable. Over the next few months, she introduced me to her school friends, Dua and Ella, who became like sisters to me. At a time when friendship groups could be so cliquey, Sarah did the opposite – generously and warmly inviting me into her life. These girls showed up through all the darkest periods, continuously inspired me, and helped to rebuild my confidence. Even when my life was the opposite of glamorous and sparkly, they made me feel that I was worth something, and that anything was possible.

Then there was Moya, who I met because we worked with the same agency. We hadn't been particularly close before I moved in with her, but she became fundamental to my recovery. She was the perfect person to have around when I was low. She never pushed me to do anything, but she encouraged me to do things that would make me feel better, such as going for runs. She rebuilt my confidence and always showed me love and empathy, especially when I needed it most.

I would be lying if I said I hadn't lost friends along the way. When you struggle with mental health, you learn a lot about people by who sticks around. In the end, it's only a positive thing, because it means everyone in your life is there for a reason. I count myself extremely lucky to have been propped up so many times, especially because family and friend support is considered to be a key factor in reducing the probability of recurring manic episodes. It's a massive privilege, but instead of feeling guilty about it, I'm trying to embrace it and make use of it. In my lowest moments, when my brain loves to tell me I'm alone, I can remind myself just how untrue this is. I can say with absolute certainty that love has got me through the worst of my bipolar.

With any relationship, whether romantic or platonic, I have realised that stability is the most important trait. With a label such as bipolar, it's easy to think a 'stable' life isn't possible. But I think you can always find something to hold on to, even in the choppiest of waters. Although my relationship with M wasn't to be, I loved that I could be some form of stability for him. After so long relying on everyone else, I loved being relied on.

Just because my moods are erratic doesn't mean I can't love and support someone else. If anything, I like to think it makes me more empathetic and understanding. When someone is having a hard day, my God can I relate. I know some of my tendencies can be challenging for anyone who loves me. But I also know what I bring to the table: the capacity for a huge amount of love.

11
my mind at work

Since being diagnosed with bipolar, my career has been a constant concern. *What should I do with my life? What can I do with my life? Will I ever be able to work alongside people again, when my brain works so differently to everyone else's?* These questions have plagued me since 2018 – and sometimes they still do, if I'm honest.

I often think about how my pre-diagnosis career contributed to my mental health. I'm not saying that modelling caused my bipolar (even though a terrible therapist did suggest this was the case), but I do think it added fuel to the fire that triggered my manic episode.

It's difficult to be 'stable' if you work as a model. You're constantly prodded and poked and endlessly judged. Every single expression you make is pored over and analysed. The career is full of highs and lows at the best of times. The highs – booking a super-cool job, or seeing your face all over billboards – are pretty hard to beat. The lows include a casting agent making a negative comment about your appearance, the rejections, or spending extended periods of time out of work. It's no wonder that my up-down personality went unnoticed during my modelling years. In a way, it was a natural part of the job.

Undeniably, my bipolar well and truly developed during my fashion heyday, even if it flew under the radar among the racks of clothes and camera flashes. I was addicted to the highs that came with my career. I would regularly have grandiose thoughts about my success as a model, believing I would become the most famous, most well-respected model in the world. It was destined, it was fate ... it was the epitome of self-belief. But then there were the waves of self-hatred and anxiety that regularly came crashing.

In the build-up to my episode, it was hard to remember why I loved modelling so much. When I was low, I felt self-conscious that I couldn't deliver that fun and vibrant person my regular clients had come to expect. I had to cancel jobs in the throes of depression, and low self-esteem was a constant struggle. Every time I was rejected, I immediately blamed my appearance and felt consumed by self-loathing. I thought, *If I can't be a good model, then who am I?*

Emerging from my manic episode in 2019, I became aware that this rollercoaster lifestyle was unsustainable. But after my failed attempts at kombucha-selling and trying to get into nursing, I needed to earn money and *do something*. My ability to work felt essential to my recovery. I craved the validation of being good at something, of being useful. I always wanted to prove to others (and mostly myself) that I could thrive with my diagnosis – that I could have a successful career and a reason to get up each day. My friends all had their own exciting paths and were doing so well. I wanted to feel part of that, even though I had no clue which direction I needed to take. In the meantime, it made sense to return to what I knew, even if it was temporary. So,

I re-signed with my agency in 2019 and carried on modelling for the next few years.

This time, thanks to my medicines and the support of my family, I knew that it was OK to just earn money and do what I could, without it becoming so all-consuming. It was scary not having any end goal in sight, but I learnt to relax a little bit. Maybe it was OK to not know what I wanted to do next? Maybe the uncertainty was all part of being a 'normal' twenty-something?

It helped that I started to find other exciting things to fill me with purpose and passion alongside modelling. There was, of course, my documentary, which lit a fire in me that I didn't know existed. And then there was Viva Fever, which also felt worthwhile. Every month or so, I created a new event to raise money for a different mental health charity. I loved producing panel talks, film screenings and supper clubs – and it was so rewarding to see how these events made a difference to small mental health charities.

I had been obsessed with organising and found production easy, in the sense that I could get an event together within just a few hours of emails. It wasn't only about the money we raised; it was also about the people who came along and felt inspired or seen. A lot of people come to our events wanting to speak to me about their experience with their mental health. I love that this community enables a safe space for people to do so.

By the time I had put on a few events with Viva Fever, I started thinking that perhaps I could carve out a career in events. So, one high morning (fuelled by three coffees), I started sharing my website with lots of companies and contacts. One great benefit of hypomania is that you can get things done without freezing or doubting yourself. In a hypomanic state, I think *anything is possible*. It gives me so much self-belief, which is generally a good thing (we'll come onto the pitfalls shortly).

On a sunny October morning, I received a text from a photographer I knew. *A brand I'm working with is looking for a freelance event producer. I can connect you if that sounds good?* I couldn't believe my luck. Everything was falling into place.

A few days later, having levelled out a little from my high, I met the brand's head of marketing for breakfast. We had a great chat, and I felt so excited when I remembered that I had actually modelled for the brand when I was living in New York. The full circle moment felt like destiny. I left the meeting sure that I had secured the role, which sent me bouncing back into a three-day high.

In this hypomanic state, I trawled back through my old Facebook albums to find a picture of me working for the brand in 2016, looking very cool and edgy. The next day, I received an email with the job details. It would be a three-month contract, mainly working across their festive events. Impulsive and excited as I was, I uploaded the old photo of me to Instagram and tagged the brand, alongside a long, emotional caption (way too keen – would not recommend).

The role got off to a flying start. I helped to pull together a couple of festive events for the brand – wreath-making and bauble painting. I was booking the talent, speaking to the venues, and developing the marketing. The events were a huge success, and it was so rewarding to watch the brand's community sip wine and chat to their friends at these wholesome activities.

My next job for the brand was to work on a twenty-four hour influencer event. This wasn't quite so positive. Essentially, the brand invited twelve content creators from London to an estate in Oxfordshire, where they could get involved in wreath-making, yoga and comedy and enjoy lovely meals. In exchange, the brand hoped these content creators would post content from the trip, featuring the brand's clothes. Sounds nice, right? Sadly, my brain had other ideas.

Something about working on an influencer event that was less focused on having fun and more about filming content and keeping up appearances sent me into an existential crisis. My vocabulary across the weekend was reduced to 'cute', 'you look amazing' and 'love the outfit!' – copying the terminology of my colleagues on the trip.

I kept thinking, *What the hell am I doing with my life? Have I really jumped from modelling to this?*

I needed more purpose. I needed to feel that I was doing something useful. With these existential thoughts dominating my mind, I felt a wave of depression come over me.

Suddenly I panicked. I was pretty sure the women I worked with thought I was a bit simple, because I was confused by everything they said. One of our tasks was to decorate the table ahead of dinner, and I felt completely unable to function. It took me about twenty minutes to lay out cutlery. I was so spaced-out and frightened by my state of mind that I kept hiding in the bathrooms, hoping the mood swings would pass. At one point, I called my mum from my car, crying and telling her I might need to leave.

It might sound dramatic, but I have come to learn that my triggers are very often quite niche. The smallest thing can tip me over the edge for no rhyme or reason. Another example is long WhatsApp messages. Something about the size of them freaks me out and can send me into a low.

I sat in the car, practising calming breathing techniques, before mustering up the courage to head back into the event and try to act normal in front of my colleagues. The head of marketing knew about my bipolar, as I had spoken to her about Viva Fever, but I assume she didn't tell the people I was working with on an everyday basis – and why would she? I would have hated it if anyone drew attention to it or made me feel weird about it. But at the same time, in the midst of a panicky crisis, I didn't know where to turn. I didn't want to seem pathetic or difficult to work with.

Instead, joining in with the 'outfit reveal' element to our night, I put on one of the brand's long flowy dresses to rejoin the group and continue my small talk. I opted for a non-alcoholic cocktail, and someone made a comment about how I wasn't drinking, which made me feel uncomfortable. My mood worsened, and my attempts to hide it got weaker and weaker. By this point, when you have sunk down into the depths, conversation can become quite difficult altogether.

The following week, back at work, I called in sick. My low had spiralled for a few days, but I was nowhere near comfortable enough with the team to be honest about needing time off for my mental health. I made an excuse about having flu symptoms, which felt like the easier route.

I'm not saying this brand lacked understanding. They may have been fine with it, but I felt too scared to ask. The problem with admitting your mental health problems in a workplace is ultimately that they hired you to do a job. No matter how empathetic or kind they are, it can still be scary to admit you're not able to do what you're expected to do. Even with all the discussions about mental health in workplaces at the moment, making an excuse about physical health feels like the safest option – one you can't argue with or misinterpret. Nobody wants a colleague to bring anything contagious into the office. Poor mental health might not be catching, but it can still be debilitating.

Once my three-month contract ended, I asked my managers how it had gone. One of them said they would love to have me back and would look into the following year's budgets. The reality? I never heard from them again. I even saw that they planned an event I'd pitched, without asking me to come on board.

Being ghosted, whether romantically or in a work environment, really stings. For months, I told myself that I was useless, no fun and incapable of working in events. I felt as if I was back at square one, still as confused as ever.

Thankfully, I received some great advice that you can't give up on your dreams based on one setback, whether you suffer from mental health problems or not. Maybe they didn't think I was right for them, but reflecting on my time working there, I don't think they were right for me either. The more you discover what you don't like to do, the more it becomes clear where you should direct your energy. I promised myself that I would never work on influencer events again, and instead turned my attention to my dream event – anything to do with music. Music has always set my heart ablaze. It always sounds incredible when I'm high, and I reach for it to pull me out of a low. I love music's power to bring people together – it's akin to a spiritual experience.

After several months looking online for events roles within the music industry, I stumbled across a company on Instagram that seemed to be doing a huge variety of work. Confidence sky high again, I managed to locate a contact email and send over my CV within a matter of minutes. In my first interview, I was honest about my bipolar and the effects it can have on my mood. But I also told them how passionate I was about music and how organised I was. I tried my best to sell myself, taking into account all the great things I could bring to the table.

Thankfully, they saw something in me and offered me the role. It would be my first permanent job since, well ... ever. I received my contract, stating that I would be working nine to five (roughly, taking into account event days and evenings), four days a week. The idea of a stable job and a clear routine, after years of so much instability and uncertainty, sounded blissful.

Within a week of receiving the offer, an email arrived from one of the company's founders. She told me she had watched my documentary. *If you would like to go for a coffee before you start work here, we are keen to support you in whatever way we can*, she wrote.

I felt instantly relieved and understood. The people in a company make such a huge difference to how you experience work when you have a mental health condition. I already felt so supported, and that was massive for me. While you can never expect other people to fully understand how you feel, my God does it feel lighter when they try.

I instantly fell in love with my job, especially the fun and upbeat energy within the office and the variety of events we got to work on. I loved that the conversations within the office were always centred around music, and I knew my insight into the industry was already growing. Within a few weeks, I began to notice the positive effects that routine had on my mood. Sleep can be a huge indicator of whether I go high or low, so getting into a consistent routine when I woke up and went to bed at similar times every night worked wonders.

At first, I was worried about the regularity of my hours and how I would be able to work around my changing moods. But I actually found this to be a massive benefit of the job. When I'm high and not working, it's so easy to chase the feeling and run around messaging people, coming up with bonkers ideas and buying crap I don't need. When I'm low, it's all too easy to crawl into bed and feel sorry for myself, isolated from the world. My routine forced me to stop overanalysing my moods and just get on with it.

I'm not talking about the most intense highs and lows – just the fluctuations and mood swings I experience on a daily basis. Sometimes, it's helpful to be told what to do, to be grounded, and to be distracted. For me personally, it helps not to think about my diagnosis all the time. And the sense of achievement I get from completing a task during a low? It's second to none. I know I sometimes have to work more slowly and be more gentle with myself, but it's nice to know it's still possible.

Working with the same people every day has been amazing. I think that having a sense of community is a major factor in keeping well. Developing meaningful relationships with my colleagues has given me so much confidence. Someone once told me that the best way to get out of depression is to get out of your own mind and into other people's. It helps me if I ask my colleagues what they have been up to – to engage in conversation with them, rather than overthinking my own moods.

Still, I have to be aware of my limits. For a few weeks at work, we had events every night and I felt a lot of pressure to stay out, socialise and drink with my colleagues. This sent me into a low that lasted for a week. I've tried to be open with my colleagues and explain why I'm always the first to leave, and why I'll usually nurse a lime soda (minus the vodka) at work socials. I hate feeling abnormal, but sometimes you have to pay a small price to feel more normal in other ways.

It can be hard to know how well I'll work when I'm high. Sometimes I'm hyper-productive and whizz through emails in record time, whereas at other times I find it hard to sit still and feel extremely restless and easily distracted. I also feel a bit on edge when I'm high at work, as if I shouldn't be there, and everyone can tell I'm up in the clouds. You'd probably get fired if you came into work while under the influence of euphoric drugs. So I feel like I'm breaking the rules when I'm sitting at my desk feeling high as a kite.

I deal with this by always ensuring I have a to-do list to keep me on track, even with the most basic things, such as sending an email. When my brain is working at a million miles per hour, I have to find ways to stay focused. I'll plug into music and make sure I get outside for a walk at lunchtime. The highs tend to leave as quickly as they arrive when I'm at work – there's nothing like an angry email from a client to send you crashing down to earth, let me tell you. Work can be a leveller, which is no bad thing.

One big challenge in the workplace is how my medication can impact my performance. Every morning, I wake up completely spaced out, so I can seem completely dozy in my morning meetings. I'll miss key details, as if I have no idea what I'm doing. For the first few months of my job, I tried to reduce my medication so I could think more quickly. But after a few days, I had a horrible sinking feeling in my chest and couldn't stop crying. I realised that I can't cope without my meds, which was scary and brought up a lot of grief about the person I once was. It made me feel weak and out of control.

Eventually, I decided to speak to my boss about this. I told her that I was aware I could seem out of it in the mornings, and I was trying my best to work around it. It felt terrifying raising this, almost as if I was making an excuse – like the dog ate my homework. However, it really helped my boss understand what I go through to manage my moods. She was more thoughtful with her language and encouraged me when I performed well. It's not always easy, but I would recommend people always tell their managers if they are on heavy medication. I know it can feel like admitting we are weak, but it also allows other people to help us. There's no shame in that.

Six months into the role, I tried again to reduce my medicines and had a positive experience. Being less medicated helped me to be better at my job, and it's thanks to this that my colleagues know me better. I'm more able to voice when I'm struggling or having weeks when I can't sleep (due to the excitement of waking up again). Making those big decisions about your care is so much easier when you don't feel the pressure to act a certain way and can just be yourself.

I've already mentioned that my hypomanic grand delusions can be a blessing. When my thoughts race at a million miles per hour, I believe I can be the best at anything I set my mind to. I know what it feels like to second-guess your abilities and be filled with self-loathing, so I'm extremely grateful for moments where my self-esteem is sky-high. Nothing beats feeling unbeatable. There are so many amazing things I probably wouldn't have done had I not been spurred on by this hypomanic confidence, such as making my documentary, messaging my favourite magazine to write an article for them, and even starting a jewellery brand alongside my job.

This is another thing that I struggle to separate from my own personality. I'm surrounded by people who have done amazing, impressive, successful things. So part of me thinks, *Why shouldn't I have this level of belief? Surely anything IS possible? ... Or is it just bipolar?*

I don't think I'll ever have the answer to that, but I have learnt a thing or two about going after your dreams. You never regret the moves you make. You never regret shooting your shot – but you do regret letting opportunities pass you by.

Grand thinking also has its downsides. It makes me careless, as I often skip over important details because I feel that everything will work out in the end (case in point: funding a documentary myself. Not a good move!). I'll dig into my highs more in the next chapter – and especially how they impact risky spending behaviour. But in the workplace, this is a specific challenge I have to navigate. I tend to find it difficult to assign meaning to something that, in my mind, just isn't meaningful. I'm constantly thinking about the bigger picture and long-term goals, but a lot of work is about getting shit done on the day to day. When I'm high, I have to make a conscious effort to respect authority and take on board other people's opinions and ideas.

Even with the most supportive colleagues in the world, I still find it difficult to open up about my mental health. It's wild that I can speak so openly about my struggles on a podcast, and even lay everything on the table in this book, but asking for a mental health day at work feels like a step too far and fills me with dread. The only time I ever asked for a day off for my mental health was when I broke up with M. It felt easier because there was a specific reason.

It's much harder to say, 'I need a day off because my brain malfunctioned after I received a long text message.' It's so ingrained in work culture to keep your head down, get your work done and not make a fuss. Struggling with your mental health without a clear 'cause', such as grief or heartbreak, feels like the ultimate definition of *making a fuss*. I'm trying my hardest to break out of that, despite the discomfort, and admit when I'm finding things tough.

Navigating my break-up while being in the office every day wasn't always easy. I was waking up at 5 a.m. every day, going to yoga classes and laughing with my colleagues for the first few weeks. But when the bubble broke, the paralysing low that followed was difficult to get through. During this period, I was working in a trendy co-working spot one day, when I experienced a sudden snap out of a high. I was on the phone to my mum, chatting away about my ex, who I was convinced was definitely still in love with me. She interrupted and told me I was being deluded. I responded by collapsing in the middle of the kitchen area, sobbing on the floor, until a stranger helped me to get up.

The next day, I felt entirely different – full of energy and in a great mood. I told my colleagues that I had struggled with my mood the day before. Saying this out loud, in a much different state, I realised how easy it can be to hide bipolar. I can keep up appearances of being cheerful and level-headed and hide the most extreme aspects of my swings. I don't think that's necessarily a bad thing. It's OK to have a separation between work and home, and to keep some parts of your mental health private. You can still be authentic and honest at work, but you get to choose how much of yourself you give away. I don't want to constantly talk about bipolar at work, but I do try to speak up and ask for help when I really need it.

A huge part of feeling restless when you have bipolar is linked to being overwhelmed. When I experience this, it often leads me to procrastinate and not be able to concentrate. When your mind is so much busier than the average person's, it's about finding ways to make you feel as calm as possible. For me, I sometimes have to do a 10 km run before work to expend my energy before reaching my desk. There have also been times when I arrive at my desk in that high – I might not be able to stop laughing and find it impossible to see the point in doing anything.

I'm really fortunate that I have such a great team and I work a four-day week, so I can use that extra day to recharge and reset. Not everyone has this kind of flexibility, but I would recommend making the most of any options available. If you can choose what time to go into the office, when to eat lunch, or how often you work from home, find routines that work for you. Even if you have a strict work structure, there are ways you can find more control and agency. Whether that's getting in early so you can get on top of things before other people arrive, or you go for a run at lunch, or you build a strong community outside of work, you can find your own coping mechanisms to integrate into your day. Focus on all the things you *can* do to feel good.

One of my biggest worries since being back in a work environment is the fear of judgement. I worry that everyone thinks I'm stupid when my brain is slow from my meds, or that I'm 'too much' when I'm high, or that I'm a fun sponge when I'm low. I deal with this by remembering that you can't control what other people think of you; all you can do is try your best. I can't control how my mind works, but I can control how I respond to it.

Most of all, I try to remind myself that work isn't the be-all and end-all. It's OK to just earn money but live for the evenings and weekends. We've all gotta do what we gotta do to get by.

So many of us are caught up in the rat race. We feel that there's so much we need to achieve, and we measure our success in terms of salaries and promotions. It's understandable, because it's how the world of work is structured. It's important to have purpose and passion, but that doesn't have to come from your job.

If my psychotic breakdown taught me anything, it's that my health is my biggest priority. My work identity will constantly shift. I love pouring my energy into work, and I still get such a buzz from the feeling of achieving something. But I know where the real work lies – keeping myself well. Remember that your well-being is worth far more than any salary.

12
riding the ups and downs

Only now, five years after my diagnosis, am I beginning to embrace the highs and lows of living with bipolar. When people ask me to describe what these swings feel like, it's hard to explain, particularly because I don't know what 'normal' highs and lows are like. After all, the rollercoaster is an inevitable part of life – everyone will experience elated moods and sad moods to varying degrees. But I'll try my best to put the bipolar undulations into words.

Let's start with the highs – otherwise known as hypomania. I'd be lying if I said this isn't the best feeling in the world. I'd liken it to the pure euphoria you experience from taking MDMA (ecstasy). I feel relentlessly positive, infectiously energised and full of hope, with love for life and the world.

I can tell when I'm hypomanic within twenty minutes of waking up in the morning. It's usually an early start – I'm up before 7 a.m. – and I notice that my senses are heightened during my first coffee of the day. The rich notes will taste like something I've never had before – pure smooth deliciousness.

> WOW, COFFEE IS AMAZING!
> My mind will begin to race with thoughts.
> *I'M THE LUCKIEST GIRL IN THE WORLD.*
> *MY LIFE IS PERFECT.*
> *I CAN'T WAIT TO START THE DAY.*
> *NO ONE IN THE WORLD IS AS LUCKY AS ME.*
> *GOD, I LOVE HAVING BIPOLAR!!!*

When this feeling comes on, I almost always head for a run. I feel so much energy flowing through me, from my head to my toes, so running is the perfect way to shake it out and enjoy the grateful thoughts. The music in my headphones sounds absolutely incredible. I can hear every note, and I feel emotional about how much creativity and beauty exists in the world. I have multiple conversations with myself (in my head): from the significance of music in my life (where would I be without it?) to the day ahead (it will be perfect, surely?), and another about how my body feels (strong and fast and just amazing!). I somehow find it easy to tune into each conversation, even though my thoughts overlap and talk over one another. Each conversation is optimistic and loving. I smile and laugh to myself, no doubt looking completely unhinged to anyone I happen to run past.

No matter how many times I have experienced a morning like this, this uplifting perspective makes me feel profoundly spiritual. *Is this a moment of awakening? Is this a message from the universe? Will life feel this perfect forever?*

It feels as if I can access a viewpoint to the universe that no one else can understand, almost like a superpower.

What also makes me laugh is that in those highs, I often convince myself that I don't have bipolar. I constantly think to myself that maybe I am just an incredibly happy person and everyone else really is quite miserable. I simply can't understand why you would ever be sad, and I find talking to anyone with negative energy very difficult in these moments. I always think that this is it: mental health mastered, never to be down again.

If I grab a coffee after my run (I usually do, given it tastes too good), I notice that people respond so well to me when I'm high. I beam at the staff and everyone in the queue, asking them so many questions and enjoying every moment of these fleeting connections. Everyone is so beautiful and sweet. Humankind is pure magic! On these days, anything that would normally stress me out is suddenly funny – it's impossible to get uptight about anything.

When I was self-employed, I had a tendency to chase this feeling. It's irresistible, in the same way partygoers might take another pill when they don't want the night to end. I'd drink five or six coffees (each one elevating the high), share countless posts on social media, call my friends and parents (all I want to do is chat, chat, chat), clean the whole flat, run multiple times a day, then go to Primrose Hill and lie on a bench listening to The Beatles.

Now that I have a desk job, that isn't always possible. I've already mentioned that the vibe of an office can easily nip a high in the bud. When my mind is occupied with emails and phone calls, I neglect the high thoughts, instead of running away with them. This isn't necessarily a bad thing, because I've already mentioned that I feel self-conscious when I'm high at work. I feel like I'm breaking the rules, and often feel embarrassed by talking about myself constantly. I have also thought recently about how easy it is to hide a high at work, when this has started happening every few weeks since reducing my medication. For friends on a night out, that high is a one-off. Looking back at my diaries, these highs really started for me around the age of sixteen. Meeting new people, sometimes acting shy ... it's not all go-go-go each time. Sometimes I'm able to relax into it a bit, and I know I have mastered no one at work noticing the euphoria I'm dealing with alongside standard office conversations.

Having said that, some highs still shock me in their extremity. One symptom that you sometimes can't keep control of is the inability to stop talking (mostly about yourself). This is a big downside of being high that I struggle with. Once, I was catching up with two of my closest friends at a café. Within two sips of the coffee (unbelievably delicious), I knew that I was high, and it became impossible to listen to what they were saying. One of my friends was trying to open up about a tough time she'd been having, and I kept butting in, giving advice she didn't ask for – or need. As soon as she finished speaking about something, I would respond by comparing her experience with my own, no matter how tenuous the connection. We all know that annoying person who endlessly talks about themselves and has no awareness of anyone else. Unfortunately, I became that person. I was even conscious of my behaviour at the time, but I just couldn't stop. It was as if I had no control over what I was doing.

Later that evening, I went for a 10 km run before messaging them both to apologise. Fortunately, they responded with kindness. I'm thankful that my friends know me well enough to understand my intentions and when my bipolar alters my behaviour. They know that there's a limit to how much I am able to control my hypomania. I can get a handle on it sometimes; I've noticed that eating first thing in the morning helps to dull it somewhat. I also try to spend time alone and write in my diary when I'm high, because I know that not everyone will understand my grand epiphanies, or want to listen to my stream of consciousness. Still, it's not always possible to separate myself altogether, nor do I always want to, so I just have to ride the high as best I can.

It's strange how quickly my appetite changes when I'm high. Physically, I feel lighter – it's the literal definition of having a spring in my step. My appetite also rapidly declines. As someone who typically eats steak about three times a week, hypomania really brings out the vegan eco-warrior. When I'm high, I can't seem to look at anything other than a vegetable or a protein bar. I've always been curious to know if other people with bipolar experience this peculiar need to be the healthiest version of themselves. Perhaps it's the opposite side of the coin that makes you crave junk food when you're low. Maybe there's a subconscious desire to be the best version of yourself when you're high, just as there's a need to self-destruct when you're already down.

In such an elevated state, my confidence is sky-high. This usually means I do things I would never dream of doing on a mellow day, such as asking for someone's number in the street, or sending an out-there DM on Instagram. There are obvious pros and cons to this. In some ways, it's liberating to be free from the low self-esteem that usually holds so many of us back. If you suddenly had the confidence to go after something you want, wouldn't you take it? On the other hand, I regret a lot of these moments when I think back on them in the cold light of day. Such as the man I found on Instagram after seeing him on a dating app. I sent him a DM saying: *Sorry if this is a bit weird! I noticed you on the app a few months before but I've deleted it haha, how are you?* Cue read receipt and no reply. Not my finest hour!

I've learnt to put measures in place to prevent myself from going too far, such as deleting certain apps, and calling my mum every time I get the urge to contact my ex so she can talk me down. But ultimately this is another part of hypomania that I find difficult to control altogether. In those moments, rogue moves seem like the best ideas ever. There's no part of my brain that steps in and says, 'Rosie, you're high. This isn't actually a good idea.'

That said, I reassure myself by trying to consider the worst-case scenario. Yes, people think I'm weird, which I suppose is an accurate representation. So far, my bold moves haven't got me in much trouble – except a bit of embarrassment. But I have been embarrassed many, many times and still lived to tell the tale – it's not the end of the world.

In my case, embarrassment is something that my friends have often had to explain to me. While I might understand that I should feel embarrassed, the reality is that it's never something that weighs over me (even if I have impulsively messaged someone). The voice in my head telling me it doesn't matter what other people think has always been stronger in my internal dialogue – which I'm grateful for, considering how many times I have to listen to it.

Of course, I'm not saying this is the case with everyone and, as I've mentioned before, there are people with bipolar who can be legitimately harmful, and the reality of this sometimes scares me. But as long as my high moments aren't causing irreparable damage or hurting other people, I'm learning to feel more OK with them. What's wrong with being a little eccentric?

A big stereotype surrounding bipolar is our relationship to money, particularly the issue of compulsive spending when experiencing hypomania. Personally, when I experience a high I believe I'm insanely talented and will inevitably find success. This belief obviously impacts my relationship with money. Why wouldn't you spend lots of money if you believed it would all come back into your account (and more) thanks to some kind of divine fate? It's like if you *knew* you had won the lottery, you would probably go on a big spending blowout before the money actually lands in your account.

This was why I spent thousands making my own documentary without giving it a second thought. I regret some of my more excessive purchases, but fortunately I've never gone so wild that it has had a detrimental impact on my life. When I started reading up about bipolar, I came across worrying stories all the time, such as the banker who invested all his money into a start-up that was never going to make it and lost everything.

This story, and others like it, terrified me right from the start, so I made a conscious effort to safeguard against overspending. I regularly move money into a separate savings account that I can pay into but I can't withdraw from. My parents have the login, which requires me to call them if I want to withdraw anything. It's great because my mum can sense when a purchase is impulsive or stems from delusion, and she always checks in with me if she feels it's the latter. It helps to have people around me who can support me in keeping my spending under control.

Another coping mechanism when I feel the urge to spend is giving myself £20 to go wild in an organic food shop. I'll buy random things such as sunflower seed butter and chocolate paleo bagels. As long as I'm spending money on things I wouldn't normally buy, it satisfies the urge for impulsive spending, while allowing me to stay in check.

I'm still learning about my main triggers for hypomania. Sometimes it seems to appear randomly. At other times, it's sad moments that can trigger it, as I've mentioned before. In those cases, it can be incredibly disorientating, often filling me with shame and guilt about my 'abnormal' reactions.

Part of the reason these moments send me high is because they disrupt my sleep. Whenever I've slept less, or had a change in routine, I notice this is a major trigger for hypomania. I'm almost always high when I have jet lag or after intense periods, such as a week-long festival. I'm not sure why, but in all my research about bipolar, this seems to be quite common. I suppose lots of people would say they can become 'delirious' on little sleep, and this can translate into full-blown delusions for those who have bipolar. I also find it harder to sleep once I'm already high, which can make the hypomania last even longer. Knowing this is a trigger for me, I now have a prescription for sleeping pills that I only take when I'm high, to help bring me down to earth again.

When I first came off lithium and started experiencing hypomania again, it scared me. What if I were to run away into the euphoric abyss and end up being sectioned again? Despite these fears, with quetiapine and my other coping strategies I feel fairly safe in the knowledge that I will never go that far. Instead, I try to enjoy the benefits that hypomania offers. Having such a profound sense of optimism is truly amazing, and I try to write down all these positive thoughts when I'm up, so I have something to refer to when I'm down. Keeping a journal is helpful for this because, when you're low, it can be so easy to forget what your brain is actually capable of. I write down all my ridiculous ideas, no matter how mad, because I love how creative I become. It reminds me of how drastically my mindset can shift, which is pretty magical.

Of course, what goes up must come down. Learning to embrace the highs has also meant learning to navigate the lows. I've experienced both since I was around sixteen – though my lows would last the entirety of a school term, whereas my highs wouldn't get as much airtime (more around holidays and when I was seeing my friends). I still find the lows much more difficult to manage. Sometimes I can spot the triggers of my depression easily. I am probably in the more sensitive bracket of people on this planet. Communication is huge for me, so a long WhatsApp message from a friend saying they're upset with me will absolutely do it. If I notice someone being distant, or not being direct, this sends me spiralling into a low. I also struggle being around other people who are going through something. I absorb other people's energy, so if someone else is low, I'm bound to descend with them. This has happened quite a lot with partners and friends. I'm a complete control freak, so when I feel I can't control a situation, it can send me west.

That said, I've come to terms with the fact that my illness will often decide when depression will rear its head. Often, there's no rhyme or reason. Everything in my life will be going well, yet I'll be curled up in bed looking at the clock, willing the day to end.

If you have experienced depression, you'll know that it feels like a dark curtain over everything. It's like everything that was once good is suddenly menacing, and you can't find the way out. My eyes feel constantly heavy, as if I'm a child who needs to cry. But alongside feeling sad, it's also a very flat feeling characterised by numbness. Days, or even weeks, pass where I just don't feel like myself. The things I would normally enjoy have absolutely no effect – coffee tastes OK, and music sounds average. It's like I'm a version of myself, but the real Rosie is somewhere else entirely.

With such negative thoughts, I come to assured conclusions that everyone finds me annoying and difficult to be around. As a result, I stop speaking, because I worry that anything that comes out of my mouth will just be a burden to anyone listening. It couldn't be more of a contrast to when I'm high and speaking at a million miles per hour. Sometimes I wonder if depression is an inevitable part of bipolar – because hypomania is so exhausting and overwhelming, it's bound to create a dip. Extremes breed extremes, so the cycle continues.

In the same way I'm completely unable to notice my delusional thoughts when I'm high, I also trust my most depressive thoughts when I'm low. I believe that I am totally alone, the only person who will ever feel like this, and no one else could possibly understand. I fixate on the idea that everyone else is living perfect, social, successful lives – and mine is beyond worse. Depression is so confusing and painful, but also boring. Your brain cycles through the same old thoughts, repeating all the things it knows will hurt you most.

It's easy for other people to tell when I'm low. I'm lifeless, my eyes are glazed over, and I barely say anything. My energy drops to rock-bottom, and I can easily sleep until the early afternoon (unlike my high self, who rises when the sun does). Thanks to my low confidence, I completely lose interest in my appearance and wear the same outfit all week long, hoping no one will notice – baggy jeans, comfy trainers and a big hoodie.

It's understandable that these depressive episodes have led to suicidal thoughts in the past. When you feel so hopeless and believe that everyone hates you, the idea of living seems utterly pointless. I'm grateful that I haven't gone to those dark places – or at least, if I do, I can pull myself out of them quickly. I think it's partly down to my family's support. It's also because bipolar means that I *do* know what it means to be truly happy and optimistic. I've bounced between these two states enough times to know that they always come and go, so I find it easier to trust that the sun will come out again. In a way, this is a major blessing of having bipolar. I have regained faith that good feelings are always around the corner, even if it feels like I'm buried in the darkest cave.

Over the years, I've developed some great coping mechanisms to help me through my depressive periods. The first is resisting the temptation to hide away and isolate myself. When I used to do this, all it did was make the depression worse. I'd spiral into believing everyone was annoyed at me for cancelling on plans, that I didn't have any friends and I was totally useless, resulting in me sinking deeper and deeper. Now, I have to force myself out of the house and keep myself busy.

Even when I struggle to speak, I try to imagine what my 'high' self would say. How would she act? How would she behave? I don't always get it right, but I've realised that the 'fake it 'til you make it' approach can actually work. It's a bit like going to the gym, even when you really don't want to. You always feel better afterwards. I also now know that surrounding myself with love is the right thing to do when I'm low. Burying myself in my own miserable energy doesn't achieve anything. I can't always get back to Happy

Rosie on my own. I have to absorb other people's positive energy, and then I can feel her returning.

My second coping mechanism involves creating clear boundaries. For example, I know that alcohol is an absolute no-no when I'm feeling low. So even if I'm going out with friends, I'll just sip a soft drink and leave early. The same applies to social media – I avoid it because I know it makes me feel terrible (it fuels the thoughts that everyone is having a great time except for me). Everyone will have their own triggers and know what makes things worse. When you're low, it's easy to self-destruct and lean into those activities as a form of self-punishment. But since hitting rock-bottom, I have felt so motivated to stay away from anything that might enhance my lows, and I actively run towards anything that makes them better.

My third coping mechanism involves keeping active. I try to run towards brighter times, both figuratively and literally. I've already spoken about how important running is to me, especially during highs. But it's even *more* important when I'm low. Even when I feel like I have absolutely no energy, I know that running can be the best thing for me. Sometimes I have to force myself by laying out my running gear next to my bed, so I can change into it as soon as I wake up. There's something about running that gets everything in my body moving – I feel like my brain rewires itself while I'm moving my feet.

I like to switch up my fitness too: booking yoga classes when I'm low, as these help me recentre, decompress and generally feel more positive. I'll often book classes in advance to help keep me accountable, usually in the morning. Forcing myself to wake up early is a good way to break a low spell, and there's something about starting my day while everyone else is still asleep that enables me to access a more positive headspace for the week ahead. It also helps to break the depressive routine of oversleeping, which has to be done. Even if you don't manage it on the first day, keep trying. All problems feel more manageable in the fresh air, rather than when you're slumped on the sofa or in bed. Getting out in nature is the golden ticket for a change of mood.

Lastly, keeping house is key for coping with the lows. On those down days, I like to deep clean my flat. I find it healing to scrub the floors and organise my wardrobe. It gives me a sense of control on a day where I feel the opposite. I know that waking up early in an almost-sterile environment, with my running clothes laid out or a class booked, will slowly start turning the cogs towards a brighter day. Rather than worrying too much about whether the low will last forever, I focus on what I *can* control: actions that make me feel safe and optimistic. You have to find what works for you, almost like a depression action plan. It's hard to come up with anything while you're in a low, so having something obvious you can revert to in these times is extremely helpful.

I'm a 'rapid cycler' – a term for people who have four or more hypomanic or depressive episodes within a twelve-month period. I find that I flip between states even more frequently. I experience depression every five to six weeks (usually for a few days), and I have highs every three weeks or so: a few days of life feeling perfect. Rapid cycling means that these highs and lows can appear immediately after one another. I can sometimes experience both states in one day.

It makes sense that I go high after a depressive state because I get so excited about seeing an improvement in my mood that it tends to escalate. It's like a shock to the system, causing a physical reaction – my heart rate literally increases, and I often have stomach issues when I'm high. It's not just about my thoughts; my whole body shifts states. On the flip side, a mood swing can come on abruptly during a high, which can feel like having a panic attack. I often need to sit down very quickly; it's almost as if someone has pressed my 'off' button and I enter into shutdown mode.

When your life is dominated by changing moods, it's natural that you start to overanalyse them. I have found that tracking my moods is the worst thing for me. About two years ago, I noticed that my depression seemed to come on stronger when I was experiencing premenstrual syndrome (PMS). I decided to download a hormone tracking app to see if it could help me manage my mood. What actually happened is that I became obsessive about following this cycle, to the point where I would label my pre-period week as a complete write-off, where I'd hide away and refuse to see friends. I've now found, especially since working in a full-time job, that staying busy and distracted is the key to not analysing my mood every day. It helps me get out of my head and into the real world. Sure, I might feel lower that week, but why should I let this mood control me? It won't be the case for everyone, but I've found that adapting to my life, rather than forcing my life to adapt to me, has worked wonders. It prevents me from pinging too high or sinking too low.

Instead of tracking, I simply respect the lows when they come, and enjoy the benefits of the highs. I try not to make my moods the centre of attention. They've had enough time in the spotlight as it is. When my most extreme moods appear, I remind myself that they all pass. A new mood will come around just as quickly as this one started. In a way, this knowledge is reassuring. It's a reminder to stop chasing some magical ideal of happiness – the lows will always come, no matter what, and that's OK. Knowing that my moods would still fluctuate even if I lived an idyllic life on a beach in Bali is actually quite grounding. It reminds me to just focus on what I can control every day, and keeps me focused on the present.

Isn't that a good lesson for everyone, bipolar or not? Everything passes. All we can do is enjoy the highs, and keep moving forward in the lows.

13
give yourself time

In summer 2023, almost five years after my diagnosis, I felt that I finally came to terms with my bipolar. I was learning to trust myself, knowing my triggers and my limits, and it seemed that I could finally experience a sense of 'normality'.

The summer started with a family holiday to Amsterdam, and M (who I was with at the time) came too. That trip felt so light and easy. I wasn't the centre of attention anymore, and neither was Lucy. For years, everyone in the family had worried about us – our depression and grief – and it felt noticeably different that we were both happier and more secure. Lucy had even met someone and was embarking on a new relationship full of love and respect for her past. Instead of revolving around our sadness, family events began to revolve around my nephew – Amii's son – Dennis, who was an endlessly cheeky and hilarious toddler. Dennis reminds me so much of my dad, in that he's seemingly always in a good mood. He's constantly laughing and dancing around to music or wanting someone to play games with him. He's also fiercely intelligent, just like his grandpa.

After spending a few days with the family, M and I booked a hotel for one night on our own. We had the most beautiful evening, watching the sunset while smoking weed from one of the coffee shops and laughing our heads off. I felt so safe and secure with him; I loved going to bed together every night, always falling asleep holding hands. Even though things didn't turn out the way I thought they would, I'm still grateful for the relationship and those moments.

During this summer, my Channel 4 documentary aired, which gave me an overriding feeling of peace. The relief that the film had impacted people's lives made me worry less about my own. I didn't know what the future of my career would look like, but I felt satisfied about everything I had achieved, and hopeful about whatever might come next.

I started to let loose a little. Before I was ill, I loved going to music festivals. I adored live music, being with close friends, having limited phone signal, laughing and dancing into the early hours and going feral for a few days. After my episode, I feared that I would never be able to return to festivals again. For so long, my biggest priority was stability. The highs of a festival, the way it takes you completely outside of your ordinary life and routine, scared me. Could it trigger another episode? Still, I decided to book a weekend festival with two of my best friends. I made a promise to myself that I wouldn't drink or take drugs; I would just enjoy this time with my nearest and dearest, listening to music.

When I arrived, I decided to trust my gut. I remembered how much I'd enjoyed festivals before the diagnosis labelled me. After so many years of being careful, I became curious about what would actually happen if I just went all in. What if, for two days, I just forgot about bipolar and mood analysis? What if I did everything I had loved doing before my life became defined by bipolar?

At 3 p.m., after setting up our tents, I had my first drink. Then I had another, then another. Then I bought a packet of cigarettes, popped a few pills and had the time of my life. I laughed so much that my face hurt. I couldn't stop dancing and felt absolutely euphoric.

I'm not condoning taking illegal drugs, but I'll be honest – it was so incredible to just let go, to feel like a 'normal' twenty-something, chasing highs with my friends rather than in my own head. Of course, I was well aware of the risks. I knew that it could lead to a week-long low, but I was willing to take the chance.

The next day wasn't great. I emerged from my tent tearful and drained, and told my friends that I just couldn't do a big night all over again. I didn't have any energy left in me. Instead, we decided to do a food tour of the festival and chat about the discoveries we made on the site and the people we'd met the night before. (I fixated on a homemade crumpet van … breaking their daily PB score by eating seven in total: four Nutella, and three with cheese.) I was low, but I was still happy. I couldn't sustain a full festival in the way I used to, but I had the most incredible time with everything I *did* manage to do, and that was enough. I had survived!

I realised that it's OK to take your foot off the gas every once in a while. Yes, I still took my meds, and I listened to my gut when it told me I couldn't push myself any further. But I strongly believe it's OK to have a blowout every so often. It's OK to say 'fuck it' to the consequences, with a clear head that you know you can cope with them when they come.

In my opinion, it's important to push yourself out of your comfort zone when you have bipolar. While running, eating well and going to bed early are great for stability, there's also something to be said for not getting too obsessed with anything. Saying 'yes' to a holiday with friends, going with the flow and skipping 'healthy' days is sometimes necessary, because it helps you understand your limits. The more you can do that, the more you learn about yourself.

With or without bipolar, your twenties are for making mistakes, having miserable days and picking yourself back up again. I don't want to waste a moment of freedom, or regret not living fully. Even though it wasn't a perfect run, that festival reminded me of my lust for life.

After the festival, I went on a group holiday with M's friends. This was another breakthrough for me, because I noticed I hadn't called my parents for almost a week. While for many twenty-somethings this is completely normal, I had been heavily reliant on my parents since my episode. I rarely went a few hours without calling my mum, let alone a few days. In many ways, an episode can make you feel like a baby again, petrified of the world and desperate to cling onto someone for dear life. The fact I hadn't spoken to them so much (and barely registered it until my mum worriedly messaged asking if I was OK) made me feel that I had finally regained my independence. I felt so safe in the knowledge that they were always there to pick me up if I needed it, but I could actually stand on my own two feet too.

Another big development was restarting therapy. After breaking up with M, I was extremely scared of relapsing, and I knew instinctively that I needed to speak to a third party about my trauma and how to move forward. It took a lot of courage to make that first inquiry, given the awful experience I had had after leaving hospital. But I realised in the first session that this woman would be a much better match for me. It was nice to admit that sometimes I really struggle, feel alone and feel weird, without creating any unnecessary worry for the people I love.

After several weeks of sessions with her, I felt I had got everything off my chest and didn't have anything else to say. So I stopped. This time, I ended therapy because I actually felt I had turned a corner, rather than feeling forced to do it. I know many people prefer to be in constant therapy, and I totally respect that, but it wasn't the path for me. As of now, I feel my other coping mechanisms are really working. The positive thing is that I know I could return to it again if I ever need the extra support, and I'm really proud of myself for overcoming that fear.

At the time of writing this, I'm still on quetiapine but I'm taking the lowest dose I've been prescribed since before I was sectioned. I've worked with my doctors to find a dose that still makes me feel in control of my moods, while being secure in the idea I won't slip into psychosis.

There's no shame in being on several medicines or taking high doses. Everyone will need a different combination or quantity – mental health is individual and unique, and so is the way we treat it.

Occasionally, someone will ask me: 'Would you ever come off medication altogether?'

My answer is, 'Absolutely not.'

I'd like to exist in the same world as everyone else. I don't want to end up on another planet again, and I know that my anti-psychotic medicine keeps me firmly rooted on this one. Medication will always be a part of my life if I want to stay well, and that's completely OK.

I share the fact that I've reduced my meds as a reminder of how much things can change. Just because you're medicated to the high heavens right now doesn't mean you'll stay like that forever. Just because you feel lost and confused about your mental illness doesn't mean you won't ever live a full life. Just because you wake up every day worrying about your moods doesn't mean that one day you'll forget to even think about your mood for hours. It's possible. It's not just your moods that change like the wind. Your whole life can change too – and for the better.

Of course, I'm under no illusion that I'm fully 'cured'. I know it would be irresponsible to say that a manic episode is totally off the cards for me. For now, I feel confident that I have a handle on the most extreme parts of my bipolar, but I'm aware that nothing in life is certain – especially not mental illness. There could be something around the corner that knocks me off my feet. And I know that I've still barely touched the sides with my understanding of my illness. I am still regularly shocked and taken aback by the unexpected ways in which my brain behaves. I'm not, by any means, saying I have it all figured out. But I know as much as I *can* know, and I'm making peace with the rest.

Recovery is a complicated, and often disorientating, process. It forces you to grow up quickly in some ways, but also pushes you back to childhood in others. You're constantly wishing for the future, looking forward to a time when you'll feel 'better' and everything will be fine, while feeling stuck by the trauma of what you've gone through. It can feel as if you're being pushed and pulled by the past and the future. You can take one step forward, then ten steps back. I'm learning to accept the unpredictability of recovery. It doesn't happen in a straight line, and you just have to trust the process.

Recovering from a mental health crisis means believing that your mind is capable of good health, even after feeling so let down by it. Recovery is extremely courageous, even though it can feel like the slowest, longest slog. It means restarting your life, feeling the fear and trying again anyway. Recovery means making difficult decisions for yourself, going where your energy is, and taking it one step at a time. It means understanding that certain situations will trigger you and bring up a state of insecurity and vulnerability. Recovery is both isolating and connecting as you navigate which parts of your story you want to share with those around you, and which moments you know are best left unsaid. It's a reminder of how strong you are on your own, and how much you need other people. So many contradictions exist at the same time.

I have learnt a lot from my journey through a mental health crisis and the winding road of recovery. First of all, it really does take a village to get through mental illness. I know that I wouldn't be here today were it not for my nurses, doctors, parents and friends. In my low moments, I felt extremely guilty for all I've put them through. I felt like a burden and was so angry at myself for not being able to drag myself out of my problems. But part of unpacking the trauma of my episode has meant acknowledging that it wasn't my fault, and that I would do the same for the people I love in a heartbeat. I have that same urge to help people, which is what drove me to make my documentary and why I'm here writing this book. It's part of the magic of being human – that so many of us want to prop each other up and help each other survive. There can be pain in that, but there's beauty in it too.

I've learnt that growth can happen slowly and suddenly all at the same time. Even when you put the work in each week – exercising, finding your own coping toolkit, taking your meds, practising self-forgiveness – you still might feel like nothing is changing. But actually, everything is helping – and one day you'll notice it has snowballed, and you'll wake up and look around and think, *Wow, I've made it to the other side of the tunnel.*

When I think back to the day I almost took my own life, lying in bed next to a drawer full of stockpiled medicines, I feel so proud of where I am today – not just staying on this planet, but *wanting* to stay.

I would never say that I 'won' the battle, and that someone else who died by suicide 'lost' the battle. I hate that idea. Our lives aren't a game. There are no winners and losers when it comes to mental health. It's insidious and unpredictable, and extremely dangerous. Siôn didn't lose anything – the world lost him. That loss – and every other loss to suicide – adds fuel to my fire to keep moving forward, and to acknowledge how quickly and seriously delusions can come. We all have a role to play when it comes to bringing the darker sides of mental health out of the shadows.

Mental health is becoming a huge conversation, yet the shame remains. We all want to come across as strong, fine and normal. I wanted this more than anyone! I was fixated on the idea of being a standard twenty-something, not 'that girl who went completely loopy, lived on a locked ward and then was put on suicide watch'. For so long, I was ashamed of my struggles and my differences. I was even ashamed of my hypomania – my immense enthusiasm and excitement for life – just because it fell outside of what is considered socially acceptable. Don't we all experience these feelings in some way? We all feel pressure to follow a certain path, or to be a specific type of person, because of what we think is 'normal' – and then we feel guilt and shame when we don't fit those moulds.

Maybe it's a cliché, but I've realised there is no such thing as 'normal'. Not a single person lives a totally 'normal' life;

everyone has something they're dealing with behind closed doors, and there's always more than meets the eye. We all have pain points and traumas, eccentricities and quirks. Our brains function in numerous weird and wonderful ways – and, thankfully, 'neurodivergence' is becoming increasingly celebrated.

I thought my bipolar was keeping me from normality – but it's actually my own version of it. Extreme highs and lows are my normal. Taking anti-psychotic medicine is my normal. Constantly trying to keep my feet firmly planted on Planet Earth – that is my normal. It might not seem normal to other people, but it doesn't need to. We all have to learn to find our own version of normality, free from what we think we 'should' be.

Accepting my bipolar has meant taking each day as it comes. Instead of focusing on a long-term goal of happiness (as so many of us do), I've shifted my focus towards tackling whichever route my brain wants to go down in a given day. I have learnt to define 'happiness' differently. It's not only about being in a state of euphoria all the time. I already know too well what would happen if I couldn't pull myself down from hypomania. Instead, I've decided that depression can even be a part of happiness. Each low period teaches me more about my brain than I knew before. Having resilience and coping with the lows helps me appreciate the highs when they come.

I'm constantly amazed by how resilient we, as humans, are. I'm reminded of that every time I look at my parents who have lost a son, and my sister who has lost a partner, and see how positive and hopeful they can be. And now, I'm reminded of it every time I look in the mirror. The lows in life are extremely painful, and I know that we all wish we could get rid of them. But it's so inspiring that we manage to go through all this shit and still survive and thrive afterwards. I think we are fundamentally an optimistic species, and that gives me a lot of hope.

For years, I wanted someone to take my bipolar away. When I first became ill, I was so angry that my seemingly perfect life had been ripped away from me. Now I wouldn't trade my up-and-down bipolar life for anything. Believe it or not, this illness has actually given me more than it has taken from me. It has taught me how resilient and strong I really am. The word 'perspective' is thrown around a lot, but I am genuinely so grateful for the most basic things, such as going to work and getting out for a run – because I know how hard it can be when the chips are down.

I believe I have become much more open-minded and empathetic, because I know that our minds are deep and scary, and you never know what's going on inside someone else's. It has made me want to make a difference in a way that just wasn't on my radar before I was diagnosed. As much as my career has been unpredictable since then (and I still don't know what the future holds), it has given me a sense of purpose.

Bipolar keeps me on my toes. It keeps me curious and wanting to learn and adapt. It reminds me that nothing is definite, nothing is certain, and we can't control everything – as much as we want to. In a lot of ways, my life did end when I was sectioned on that hot September day. But a new life started. It was difficult at first, but I think I prefer the new Rosie.

I believe that bipolar is my spark. It's what makes me who I am. Feeling the depths of emotion can be exhausting but it's also magical. I'm reminded every day of how powerful my mind can be – how powerful *all* our minds are. They can be cruel and crippling, as well as bright and inspiring. Bipolar brains are a force to be reckoned with. I wish I knew that when I was twenty-two.

A few years ago, I read countless books that told me my life would be chaotic forever. And here I am, finishing writing my own book while listening to classical music in complete stillness. At peace with my past, and excited about my future. I hope that no matter how 'abnormal' your mind seems, you'll eventually come to a place where you accept it and respect it – and even enjoy the journey.

OUR VOICES

A huge part of my recovery came after meeting other people with bipolar. Those interactions reminded me that I am not alone in this, while also teaching me that you can never compare your journey to someone else's. I wanted to include a few people's experiences after my own to conclude this book.

Luyando Malawo
Instagram: @livingwithluyando

'I was diagnosed with bipolar type 1 in 2014 when I was twenty-four years old. I was sectioned, and then diagnosed when I was discharged. I would describe my highs as experiencing unfiltered optimism. Everything seems easily achievable: all my ideas are great. I feel like I'm floating and gliding through life and think I can do multiple things at once. I'm quick-witted, funnier and more creative. However, when I had my first full-blown manic episode, it was terrifying as it escalated to psychosis. Thank goodness that has only happened once.

'I'm not exactly sure what triggers my highs – it can be a lack of sleep, and I certainly feel a shift and lift in mood after every monthly menstrual cycle. I cope with them by trying to slow down and rest. I also make sure I keep my plans realistic!

'My lows, on the other hand, feel terrible. I'm angry, irritable, lethargic and have a negative, hopeless outlook. My triggers include conflict, overwhelm and when I feel like I've failed at something. Alcohol can be a trigger too. It depends on the severity, but sometimes a good night's sleep helps me reset, talking to a friend and confronting tasks I've been dreading or find challenging. I always go to therapy or call a mental health helpline when I'm having concerning thoughts or feelings.

'This is what I'd say to someone who has been recently diagnosed: "Congratulations on the new chapter of your life. A lot now can be explained and helped. Embrace it, and let this new diagnosis mean well for you."'

Aparna Piramel Raje
Instagram: @aparnapiramalaraje

'I live with bipolar 1. My manic episodes started in 2000 when I was twenty-four, but I only got an official diagnosis much later in 2013 when I was thirty-seven. This was due to a bunch of reasons – mainly concerns about medication, and discomfort about the 'label' of bipolar. I've now been on medication since 2013.

'My highs are exhilarating and sometimes traumatic. I feel alive as never before, and extremely creative. I don't sleep much, but I'm consumed by my thoughts and writing five times as much as normal. Some of it is pretty good. If I ascend into mania from hypomania, I start losing control of my mind, and if I'm psychotic, that can get a bit scary.

'My highs are usually triggered by a combination of interpersonal conflict and work-related stress. Also anger against social injustice – of which there is so much in the world! Once I take something to help me sleep, I'm much more in control. In addition, yoga, walks, gym, cleaning out my cupboards, spending time with my family all help me to come back to base camp.

'I always say that mania is tough on my family, while depression is tough on me. My lows usually follow immediately after my highs. I'm consumed by feelings of hopelessness, despair, worthlessness manifested in being quiet, withdrawn and lethargic.

'I'm able to cope better with my lows because I tell myself that this is not me – this is not who I am. I generally see myself as a warm, optimistic, caring person so I'm able to step back from the low and detach. Support from friends and family is really important, as is giving myself enough time to heal and recover from a manic episode.

'It is completely possible to live and thrive with a mental health condition. Bipolarity for me has been my guru, my source of inner illumination. I've learnt so much about empathy, resilience, courage, gratitude and mindful detachment. So let your vulnerability teach you what it can teach you … and you can live the life you dream of.'

April Kelley
Instagram: @april_kelley

'I have type 2 bipolar and was diagnosed in March 2018. My highs can only be described as euphoria. A day(s) release from my mind. Anything is possible. No need for sleep. I'm intoxicating to others and toxic to myself. It makes me feel like I'm cured or that I'll never have a low again, but over the years I unfortunately know that'll never be the case. That's something I have to come to terms with.

'Lack of sleep (be that from work or socialising too much), meeting new people and success at work all trigger my highs. My friends and family tend to notice when I am high before I do, which is a massive help.

'In my lows, I'm extremely anxious and paranoid. There are thoughts of suicide. Feeling hopeless and worthless. Some lows simply just occur, and I can't figure out why; I can only presume it's the chemical imbalance at work. And there are lows that are brought on by people. It could be a small thing and it'll throw me into an episode.

'I can pull myself out of a low by sleeping as much as possible. Have reminders to eat. Allow myself a day in front of the TV to escape. Do some sort of activity or sport if I can get myself to leave the house. Most importantly, I've learnt to give myself something to look forward to every day. Whether that's something bigger like a gig or a day trip, or something small like ice cream, I just make sure I have something to look forward to.

'I'm a rapid cycler, and some of my symptoms can signal a high or a low, so it can be hard to differentiate which direction I'm going into. My sleep pattern is the biggest signal, and sleep is the biggest coping mechanism for me.

'I would say this to someone who has just been diagnosed: "You're safe. The diagnosis is a lifeline. You've been fighting the demon in the dark. A diagnosis turns the light on, so now you, and your loved ones, can see what you're fighting."

'When I told my dad about my diagnosis, before anything else he said, "I always knew you had a spark of genius." I believe that to be true of anyone living with bipolar. You have a spark of genius.'

James Harrop
Founder of @theminderfulworld

'I was diagnosed with bipolar disorder type 1 when I was twenty years old. When I'm high, it feels like reality breaks down. I'm stuck between two worlds: one created by my accelerated thoughts, full of meaning, trying to make sense of what is happening; and the other world, where everyone else operates. As I go deeper, or higher, into the high, delusions creep in. Time becomes meaningless; I am no longer in the flow of life – I *am* the flow of life. It all gets weird, very weird, until eventually my hand is forced and I require help.

'I can spin into mania if I don't take my medication consistently – and then, through lack of sleep, I'm drawn powerlessly down the well-trodden paths back to mania and delusion; always thinking, *This time it is different; I can control it.*

'Daily medication is the biggest helper. Secondly, no stimulants. Thirdly, recognising that the highs are part of the illness. And my support network is the greatest help of all.

'For whatever reason, my lows are not nearly as intense as my highs. The self-critical voice is dialled up loudly, most noticeably self-loathing and a feeling of uselessness. This can be triggered by alcohol, lack of exercise, and a life that becomes monotonous or lonely.

'A broad and diverse wellness routine helps to pull me out of my lows, which includes cardio exercise, eating healthily, getting sufficient sleep, not drinking excessively, practising yoga, meeting with friends, engaging in breathwork, drinking plenty of water, boxing or weight training, and surrounding myself in nature.

'My message to any new members of the bipolar club? "The wind of the Universe never harms you." And, "Take your meds."'

ACKNOWLEDGEMENTS

Amanda, Victor, Amii, Lucy, Sarah, Dua and Ella for holding me through grief.

James, Dennis and Elliott for your continued love.

Rosa, Alicia, Maddie, Sophie, Shamus, Azure, Sophie and Moya for being my backbone every single day.

Poppy, Marni, Indya and Ella for helping me build Viva Fever with such kind hearts.

Grace and Sophie for restoring my confidence in my career and encouraging me to reach my potential.

Mireille and Arielle for allowing this book to exist and reach the world in a way which feels Rosie.

Siôn, for the fire in me which pushes me to talk (very) loudly about mental health.

A NOTE ON THE AUTHOR

Rosie Viva is a model, documentary filmmaker and activist passionate about encouraging and helping people talk about neurodiversity. 2023 saw Rosie become the subject of a Channel 4 digital documentary, *Modelling, Mania and Me*, charting her day-to-day experiences of living with bipolar which has amassed over 100,000 views since May 2023. Channel 4 want to make Rosie the channel's next 'face of mental health'. An ambassador for Bipolar UK, Rosie's writing and work has been featured in *Grazia*, *Stylist*, *Women's Health*, *The Telegraph*, *BBC*, *Daily Express* and Dua Lipa's *Service95* newsletter, and has recently appeared on *Steph's Packed Lunch* as well as on BBC Radio London and Gurl's Talk.

A NOTE ON THE TYPE

The text of this book is set in Linotype Sabon, a typeface named after the type founder, Jacques Sabon. It was designed by Jan Tschichold and jointly developed by Linotype, Monotype and Stempel in response to a need for a typeface to be available in identical form for mechanical hot metal composition and hand composition using foundry type.

Tschichold based his design for Sabon roman on a font engraved by Garamond, and Sabon italic on a font by Granjon. It was first used in 1966 and has proved an enduring modern classic.